Doctors Re-examine Circumcision

Thomas J. Ritter, M.D. and George C. Denniston, M.D.

Copyright © 1992, 1996, 2002
by Thomas J. Ritter and George C. Denniston.

Formerly titled, *Say No to Circumcision:*
40 compelling reasons why you should respect
his birthright and keep your son whole.

All rights reserved. No part of this book may
be reproduced in any form without written
permission from the publisher.
Printed in the United States of America.

ISBN 0-9711878-0-0
(previously ISBN 0-934061-30-0)

To purchase this book, write:
NOCIRC – PA
P.O. Box 103
Mountville, PA 17554
MusiciansUnited@aol.com
Or call (717) 285-2839

Third Millennium Publishing Co.
2442 NW Market St. #42
Seattle, WA 98107

London; New York; Mt. Vernon, Iowa; Seattle

Dedication

For AWN, who started me on this crusade.

"I am a general surgeon. The prime dictum in medicine is "Thou shalt do no harm." The intent of this book is to explode the myth that routine newborn circumcision does no harm."

Thomas J. Ritter, M.D.

Acknowledgments

This book has already been helping parents make an important decision for seven years. Under normal conditions, this book would go out of print. But the demand for the book persists. Under a new publisher, and with some significant revisions, including the title, this book is again seeing the light of day.

Our thanks to the original publisher, Ken Albert, for supporting a pioneering effort, and for his generosity. We thank Robert Van Howe M.D., a pediatrician and internationally respected expert, for his suggestions and additions. We thank Lisa Stephon of NOCIRC-PA for her commitment and support of this revised version. As the distributor, she will make it possible for thousands of new parents to learn about this practice before it is too late.

A message to parents who were responsible for their son's circumcision

If you were responsible for your son's circumcision, the information in this book will make you sad, and angry, and it will fill you with regret and guilt. Please don't be defensive. And please don't say, "It would be better if everybody would just be quiet. It's too late now anyway."

No, it's not too late. Let's think about child physical and sexual abuse, in general. Are people wrong to speak out about child abuse? Of course not. It's the only way to raise awareness, to change our laws and institutions so that these crimes against innocent children are not perpetuated generation after generation. Speaking up will break the cycle.

The same is true of circumcision. Concerned people must speak out so that this harmful, abusive practice is stopped. And besides, the circumcision you feel responsible for wasn't your fault. You didn't know the truth—maybe your doctor didn't even know the truth. All you can do is apologize. Tell your son you're sorry. And then talk with other parents and friends so they know that a natural penis is the best penis.

To new parents

If you have any doubts that you should leave your newborn son's little penis alone, please read this book. In 1971, the American Academy of Pediatrics stated, "There are no absolute indications for routine neonatal [newborn] circumcision." This means that the doctors who are responsible for children's well-being have officially opposed routine circumcision for over 20 years.

Please do not just hope that you will have a girl, so that the issue will not arise. Please have the courage to let your son decide for himself. Protect him from infant circumcision. Be aware of the bias that a circumcised doctor may have in caring for your intact son's penis. Refuse to permit doctors to circumcise him as an infant or as a boy for whatever "reasons" they may come up with. Beware of doctors who forcibly retract your son's foreskin. Warn them *in advance* not to do so.

Be sure to tell your boy that he is normal, and fortunate. Have him understand that it is others who have had a normal part of their body removed without their consent. If he asks you why, you may have difficulty, because no one knows why! You may find part of the answer in this book. What are the indications for operating upon, and removing, a normal structure?

When he reaches the age of maturity, let him decide for himself whether or not he wishes part of his normal penis to be removed.

We have the greatest admiration for fathers who, having been circumcised themselves, refuse to permit their own sons to be circumcised.

A special message to circumcised men

The message of this book is clear. Circumcision has no medical purpose. And even more compelling, it diminishes the male penis. This is not information that any circumcised man wants to read or acknowledge.

Obviously, the penis is a key sex organ. Men couldn't have sex without it. But there is another organ in the body that overwhelms the sexual power of the penis. You're right, it's the brain. And nobody has a circumcised brain, so everybody can still have a fulfilling sex life.

And there is an even happier message for circumcised men. There are ways you can restore your foreskin, if you choose (see Chapter 20). Some methods require some time and effort. Others are quicker but more expensive. But be assured, there are solutions. So fathers, don't circumcise your baby sons to look like you. Rather, if you're motivated, restore your foreskin so you can look like and function like your intact son when he grows up.

A message to doctors who circumcise

It should interest you to know that you are violating the Golden Rule (would you have wanted someone to do this to you without your permission?); the major tenet of medical care, First, Do No Harm; and all seven Principles of The American Medical Association Code of Ethics.*

We have come to a turning point with respect to circumcision. With the publication of this book, Dr. Jim Bigelow's book, *The Joy of Uncircumcising*, and the growing influence of NOCIRC and NOHARMM, the word is out. No longer will excuses suffice for performing neonatal circumcision. Doctors, from now on, will be held accountable. They may no longer use their licenses to remove normal tissue, which is not in the best interests of their patient, without paying a penalty.

U.S. medical policy in 2001

The American Medical Association (AMA) made its first statement on circumcision on July 6, 2000.

"The AMA supports the general principles of the 1999 Circumcision Policy statement of the American Academy of Pediatrics (AAP), which reads as follows:" (see below)

Council on Scientific Affairs, AMA, *Neonatal Circumcision*, July 6, 2000

The American Academy of Pediatrics based its recent policy statement on a review of the past 40 years of scientific papers on the topic.

"Existing scientific evidence demonstrates potential medical benefits of newborn male circumcision; however, these data are not sufficient to recommend routine neonatal circumcision."

If the data are not sufficient, then clearly the harm outweighs the "potential medical benefits." The procedure has insufficient medical reasons. Therefore a doctor cannot perform it.

(continuing AAP statement) "In circumstances in which there are potential benefits and risks, yet the procedure is not essential to the child's current well-being, parents should determine what is in the best interest of the child. To make an informed choice, parents of all male infants should be given accurate and unbiased information and be provided the opportunity to discuss this decision. If a decision for circumcision is made, procedural analgesia should be provided."

American Academy of Pediatrics Task Force on Circumcision. Pediatrics 1999; 103(3): 686-693

Can a doctor provide adequate informed consent, and can parents legally give consent for their son's penis to be partially amputated? Legal opinion now says no, they cannot.

…reliable information regarding the surgery is not usually made available to parents when they are asked to consent to the procedure for their newborn sons…many medical professionals, medical ethicists and legal scholars now dispute the advisability, and even permissibility, of circumcising newborn boys…a prominent Canadian medical ethicist recently went so far as to assert that neonatal circumcision constitutes assault under the Canadian criminal code….numerous legal scholars have concluded that routine neonatal circumcision falls within the legal definition of child abuse and violates children's civil and human rights under national and international law. Consent to a procedure that is per se illegal is, of course, invalid regardless of the motives of the consenting party. But even if it were legally and ethically permissible for parents to authorize circumcision of their sons, empirical studies have shown that the manner in which doctors typically obtain "informed consent" for neonatal circumcision from parents falls far below the standard of care required of the medical profession *…because routine circumcision causes significant harm while providing no appreciable medical benefits, parental consent to the procedure is invalid.* If circumcision can ever ethically and legally be performed, it is only when the male reaches adulthood and is capable of deciding for himself to undergo the procedure.

Svoboda, JS, Van Howe RS, Dwyer JG. Informed Consent for Neonatal Circumcision: An Ethical and Legal Conundrum. Journal of Contemporary Health Law and Policy. 2001; 17:61-133

---

*Denniston, GC. Circumcision and the Code of Ethics. Humane Health Care International 1996;12(2):78-80.

Preface

George C. Denniston, M.D.

When you finish reading this book, you will no longer favor circumcision for your tiny newborn son. After all, you would not dream of circumcising your daughter, or a puppy. Why is it all right to circumcise your son?

The United States is the only country in the world that circumcises half its newborn sons. Fifteen years ago, almost 90% of American newborns were circumcised. Now the numbers are running just over 50%. Millions of American parents have chosen, and are choosing, not to circumcise.

Doctors have tried to say it is the parent's decision. Modern medical ethicists say that parents can make decisions for their child *"only if these decisions are in his best interest.*

Nothing supports the notion that circumcision is in the best interest of the child. It removes a healthy, normal, useful body part. Rarely does this part need to be removed for medical reasons. Virtually all the alleged medical reasons are invalid. In Finland, where the intact penis is valued, no one is circumcised at birth, and only one in 16,667 is circumcised later in life.* The foreskin is very normal indeed, and can invariably be cared for without surgery, but only by persons who are determined to preserve the intact penis.

It is harmful to men to have their foreskins removed at birth. Hundreds of men have now come forward, and have testified to that fact in writing.

The foreskin has useful functions. It protects the glans penis throughout life, it covers the shaft of the penis, which enlarges when it erects, and it provides sexual sensitivity that is destroyed when it is missing.

As a parent, you would not want to harm your son, or remove a useful part of his sexual anatomy. But even if you should still want to do this, no doctor should want to participate. Here is why: There are no valid medical reasons for performing circumcisions, only excuses. The risks and disadvantages of circumcision far outweigh any possible protective benefits. Any doctor who tells you otherwise is misinformed about relative risk. A doctor who performs circumcisions is violating the Golden Rule - if he were intact, he would not permit this to be done to himself, without his permission. He is violating the major tenet of medical practice, First Do No Harm. Last, but not least, he is violating *all seven Principles* of the AMA Code of Ethics.

A doctor performing circumcision today usually removes far more tissue from the penis than was removed during the period of both the Old Testament and the New Testament. During Biblical times, only the tip of the foreskin was removed. Today the foreskin is removed at the base of the glans, for no medical reason. Circumcision has suffered an escalation from the original Biblical injunction, advocated by mere mortals, with tragic consequences.

Circumcision is not surgery, by definition. In his classic *History of Surgery*, Welch has defined surgery to include: repair of wounds, extirpation of diseased organs or tissue, reconstructive surgery, and physiologic surgery (e.g., sympathectomy).** Routine newborn circumcision eludes classification. If it is not surgery, what is it?

Obstetricians should not do circumcisions. They are operating on a pediatrician's patient, without prior consultation. Also, males are not supposed to be patients of this specialty, according to the American College of Obstetricians and Gynecologists.

Pediatricians certainly should not perform circumcisions. Their entire commitment is to *protect* the child.

Urologists rarely have medical justification for removing foreskin. It robs the organ of their specialty of too many functions.

Family physicians will cease to perform circumcisions, because they will no longer wish to violate the ethical basis of their profession.

Many doctors who do not really believe in circumcision still perform it under pressure from colleagues, hospitals, and parents. Doctors who do not approve of circumcision ought not perform them. Doctors who stop performing circumcisions certainly are to be admired.

Parents will not do it. Doctors will cease to do it. What is left but to permit the young American male to grow up intact and enjoy his sex life as a whole, intact person?

If anyone still persists in circumcising, let us understand why this might be:

If this person is male, he has been cut, and is in denial. He has not yet mustered the courage to say, "They did it to me, but I am not going to do it to my son! (or my patients!)"

If this person is female, she has agreed to circumcisions and may be saying to herself, "This is the one thing about my son's birth I truly wish I could take back." But she cannot, and is having a hard time accepting that. Millions of American mothers fervently wish they could undo the circumcisions they unwittingly authorized.

The strong denial mechanism that humans have may be why circumcision has persisted. Once understood, it will cease to cause harm to future generations.

---

*Wallerstein, E. *Circumcision: An American Health Fallacy*. New York: Springer Pub Co., 1980.

**Welch, L S. The History of Surgery in David L, ed.: *Christopher's Textbook of Surgery*, ed. 8, Philadelphia, 1964, W.B Saunders Co, pp. 1-23.

Foreword

It is a remarkable fact that there hardly exists a people in the world that does not, in one way or another, mutilate its members. There is hardly a part of the body that has not been the object of what, to the dispassionate observer, would appear to be the calculated wrath of its elders, for it is usually upon the young, and frequently the newborn, that these mutilations are inflicted. Homo sapiens, "the wise guy," in the name of reason behaves in the most irrational manner, and commits the most atrocious of cruelties upon the bodies of his victims, and sometimes upon his own. Such acts are usually justified by programmatic myths and rituals, as well as by rationalizations which serve to "explain" the reason for such practices. The functional role of myths is to provide a sanction for a course of action. Myths in the course of time become comfortable realities. Ritual invests them with importance, and renders them sacred. The myth and ritual of circumcision are of epidemic proportions, in the United States more than in any other civilized country.

The monstrous myths that have captivated men's emotions and shackled their minds, still afflict the minds of millions in so-called civilized societies. The ambiguities and uncritical use of our language gives rise to ambiguities of their own, and constitute the compost upon which myths proliferate and are sustained. In the reality which every society creates for itself the unreal becomes more real than the real, so that myths become quite unaccountable to any other reality, developing as they do, an integrity, a validity, and a power, which is quite impregnable to any attempted demonstration of the unreliability of their component parts. It is of the nature of myth that it is elaborated, but never proved. But this doesn't mean that myths cannot be disproved. They can. We realize that people have different investments in their beliefs, that humans are governed more by custom and precedent than by logic and reason, that errors and illusions which serve some explanatory purpose frequently become endemic myths shared in common in the world of unreason and political fantasy. Myths that at one time may have served a socially useful purpose, may perpetuate themselves into a time when they have become not only useless, but thoroughly baneful, decayed and degraded.

It is to this challenge, presented by the widely pervasive myth of circumcision in the United States, that Dr. Ritter has magnificently responded in this fascinating and highly readable book. As a physician and surgeon of considerable experience, and a deep understanding and knowledge of what circumcision is, its history, development, secular, religious, and medical implications, Dr. Ritter is one of the first medical authorities to have taken a strong stand against the practice of circumcision. His book is extraordinarily good because it is written by a warm, humane, and very knowledgeable person, who very deeply cares for people, and especially babies, the principal victims of this archaic practice. Since circumcision is so ancient a practice, and has been widely ritualized in the United States, Dr. Ritter has set out to show how the practice originated, how it has been sustained by religious groups, and only too often by the very profession that should have been the first to protest against the practice, his own. What is so especially valuable about this book is that Dr. Ritter musters all the facts which show beyond equivocation how damaging, from every point of view and consideration, circumcision is. He shows beyond dispute how erroneous, and indeed, how damaging in their effects, are the medical claims for circumcision, all this supported by a full and convincing array of the evidence, many illuminating tables and illustrations, which together make the best, and quite unanswerable case against circumcision that, to my knowledge, has ever been written. It is an achievement for which all of us should be grateful, and most of all the babies and their parents.

Ashley Montagu, Ph.D.
Internationally acclaimed anthropologist & author
Princeton, New Jersey

Some of the Fallacies and Myths of Circumcision

- Circumcision is necessary.
- Circumcision is not painful or traumatizing.
- Circumcision prevents disease.
- The circumcised penis is cleaner.
- The circumcision decision is up to the parents.
- Men don't mind that they are circumcised.
- A circumcised penis is as good or better than a natural penis.
- Circumcision has little or no surgical risk.
- Complications are rare in circumcision surgery.
- The uncircumcised penis is difficult to care for.
- The foreskin is extra skin, a mistake of nature.
- A penis with a foreskin looks unnatural.
- A circumcised penis provides just as much sexual pleasure.
- Circumcision removes just a snip of skin.
- A son should "look like" his father.
- Everyone is circumcised.
- He should be circumcised to "fit in" the locker room.
- Circumcision prevents masturbation.
- Circumcision is necessary to prevent cancer.
- Circumcision prevents urinary tract infections.
- Circumcision prevents the spread of sexually transmitted diseases, including AIDS.
- You can rely on your doctor's advice on circumcision.
- Circumcision prevents premature ejaculation.
- He'll just have to have it done later.
- All doctors endorse circumcision.
- Insurance will pay for it.
- It didn't harm me. My penis is fine.
- Christians should be circumcised.
- Jews don't question circumcision.
- The foreskin should retract at birth.

Victims' Voices Note

Actual letters and statements of real people who have and are suffering the abuses of circumcision are included in this book. Initials and locations have been changed to protect their privacy.

Contents

1	Circumcision Inflicts a Diminished Penis on Your Newborn Baby Boy	1-1
2	Circumcision Is Really Foreskin Amputation, and Is Abusive	2-1
3	Circumcision Is Very Painful and Traumatizing—A Terrible Way to Welcome Your Newborn	3-1
4	Circumcision Produces Psychological and Emotional Pain and Anguish to Sons and Parents	4-1
5	Circumcision Creates Unnecessary Surgical Risks and Complications	5-1
6	Cleanliness and Hygiene Reasons Mandate That We Do Not Circumcise	6-1
7	No Extra Care Is Needed for an Intact Infant or Young Boy	7-1
8	Your Son Will Learn How Simple it Is to Keep Himself Clean	8-1
9	The Foreskin Is Normal and Natural	9-1
10	What Looks "Funny" to Some Is Natural and Normal	10-1
11	When Unaroused, the Glans of the Penis Is Meant to Be an Internal Organ, Like the Clitoris	11-1
12	The Foreskin Enhances Sexual Pleasure!	12-1
13	Circumcision Robs the Male of His Birthright—A Fully Functioning Penis	13-1
14	It Makes Just as Much Sense to Circumcise Baby Girls	14-1
15	Circumcision Is a Disservice to Both the Male and Female—Especially in Later Life	15-1
16	Europeans and Asians Do Not Circumcise Their Sons	16-1
17	The "I'm Circumcised and I'm Fine" Syndrome	17-1
18	Circumcision Removes A Lot More Than a Little Snip of Skin	18-1
19	Your Son's Penis Does Not Have to Look Like His Father's	19-1
20	Men Circumcised as Infants Are Even Now Restoring Their Foreskins	20-1
21	Males with Foreskins Will Have A Lot of Company in the Locker Room	21-1
22	Males Masturbate Whether They Have Foreskins or Not	22-1
23	The History of Circumcision Is Filled with Hysteria, Bias, Misinformation, etc.	23-1
24	Christianity Does Not Require or Promote Circumcision	24-1
25	Some Jewish People Are Even Changing Their Minds on Circumcision	25-1
26	Don't Be Fooled, Most Books, Including Medical Textbooks, Contain Inaccurate Information	26-1
27	Don't Accept, at Face Value, What Your Doctor Has to Say About Circumcision	27-1
28	Most Physicians Are Circumcised Males' or Female Doctors Whose Husbands or Sons Are Circumcised	28-1

Contents
(continued)

29	Make No Mistake, There Is Money in Circumcision	29-1
30	Circumcision Does Not Prevent Premature Ejaculation	30-1
31	Penile and Cervical Cancer Are Not Valid Reasons for Infant Circumcision	31-1
32	The Intact Penis Is Not More Prone to Urinary Tract Infections	32-1
33	The Intact Penis Is Not More Likely to Spread STD's, Including AIDS	33-1
34	No, He Probably Won't Have to Have it Done Later Anyway	34-1
35	Intact Men Are More Likely to Use a Condom	35-1
36	Major Medical Associations Say Circumcision Is Unnecessary	36-1
37	Some Insurance Companies Are No Longer Paying for Routine Infant Circumcision	37-1
38	Many Noted Physicians and Others Have Spoken Out Against Circumcision	38-1
39	If You're Not Sure—Don't Do It!	39-1
40	Say No to Circumcision!	40-1
	Glossary	40-2
	Physician's Guide to the Normal (Intact) Penis	40-3
	Notes and Selected Medical References	40-8
	Infant Circumcision Surgery in Photos	40-9

1. Circumcision Inflicts a Diminished Penis on Your Newborn Baby Boy

Over the years, as a normal male, and as a physician and surgeon, I have always maintained a healthy interest in sexual matters. At some time in my youth, I encountered the concept, and then the reality of circumcision. The word circumcision intrigued me principally because it carried a sexual connotation—which at the time I did not fully understand. I eventually discovered that circumcision involved some type of permanent alteration of the end of the penis, but the idea still was vague and rather meaningless until I actually saw a circumcised penis. Then the spectacle was disquieting.

The permanently exposed glans, on public view, in a non-sexual setting, simply seemed inappropriate. The only time that I saw my own glans was when I was washing, urinating, or masturbating; I had a gut feeling that glans exposure only should occur in a private, personal environment. The lack of the mobile skin sheath, that normally protects and stimulates the glans, really bothered me. In my naivete, I wondered how one with this barren, sanitized penis masturbated. I wondered too why anyone would want this done to himself or why one would do it to someone else.

I already had discovered the merits of the foreskin, and I knew it was an item that I would not care to lightly cast aside. The altered penis impressed me as an inferior plaything.

Whether people wish it or not, sexual feelings are programmed into all of us. This happens to the exclusion of religious or moral standards. Certainly, sexual congress should be modified by mature, responsible social and moral conduct, but sexual functioning and/or awareness is instilled into every human being intuitively, even prior to birth. Penile erections are evident on sonography in the last trimester of pregnancy. Erections occur immediately after birth, especially associated with a full bladder. The infant—male and female—soon locates the genitalia and discovers that touching produces pleasure. Some type of masturbation is normal in all infants and children.

Each morning of their lives, most males awaken with a full bladder and an erect penis. The male holds and peruses his penis five or six times daily while urinating. He is conscious of the permutations in penile size and the pleasure associated with penile engorgement. In adolescence, erections may occur unassociated with any lascivious thought or touch, and sometimes the erection presents a social embarrassment. Sexual dreams and nocturnal emissions occur, guaranteeing that the male knows the pleasure of intercourse and orgasm, even though he may never have masturbated nor seen nor touched a female. And eventually every male child learns to masturbate. He discovers the sensitive glans and is aware that repetitive touching produces increasing sexual pleasure culminating in orgasm. Sexual indoctrination then is an exceedingly necessary, normal biological phenomenon. Nature leaves little to pure chance. Sperm must be brought into contact with the female's egg. The male has rehearsed his act and knows what to do to accomplish this. While the vast majority of human intercourse is for recreation and not for procreation, the prime purpose of intercourse still remains the perpetuation of the human race. In a biological sense, intercourse is an amoral act! In the throes of sexual arousal, rational thinking and morality go out the window. This all powerful amoral sex drive is best epitomized by a philosophic quote of one of my friends: "A stiff prick has no conscience." Nature must get the job done.

In my youth, certain aspects of male genital anatomy puzzled me: What was the function of smegma? Why was the glans asymmetric and not completely round like the cap of a mushroom? What purpose did the frenulum serve? What were the multiple, tiny, raised, purple-red hemispherical nodules concentrated especially about the corona? Why did the erecting penile shaft bow

---

- *The pertinent issue . . . is the unthinkable amputation of the normal foreskin by the vast majority of American parents.*

- *The altered penis impressed me as an inferior plaything.*

- *When one subtracts from a unit, what remains is less than the unit.*

- *"You can see a lot just by watching."*
  Yogi Berra

- *"Minor surgery is one that is performed on someone else. Using the surgical treatment of circumcision to prevent phimosis is a little like preventing headaches by decapitation. It works but it is hardly a prudent form of treatment."*
  Eugene Robin, M.D.
  Stanford University

1. *(continued)*
Circumcision Inflicts a Diminished Penis on Your Newborn Baby Boy

- *Most Americans have never seen nor experienced a sexually functioning foreskin.*

- *The masquerade that the circumcised penis is as good as, or possibly better than the normal structure, must end.*

- *Practically never can the patient, the parent, nor the physician give a sound reason for the performance of the operation (of circumcision).*

- *I want to move the American parent and male off their false base of complacent acceptance of this desensitizing, defunctionalizing operation of circumcision.*

- *"Often the less there is to justify a traditional custom, the harder it is to get rid of it."*

  Mark Twain

downward whenever the glans was uncovered by retracting the foreskin towards the body? Over the years, I succeeded in untying these sexual Gordian knots, not in one fell swoop, but by a gradual unraveling.

The contemplation of these representative sexual enigmas did not pass without a lesson being learned; what precedes, occurs simultaneously, or follows a function, often impacts critically upon that function. Modifying influences can be remote from the more obvious central issue. In one's evaluation of any unknown, it might be judicious to withhold judgment until all the facts, peripheral and central, are known. The pertinent issue under consideration is the unthinking amputation of the normal foreskin by the vast majority of American parents.

The operation of routine, infant circumcision of males involves a paradox of absurdities completely at variance with sound medical—surgical—legal practice; a normal structure is operated upon; no anesthesia is used; the patient does not give his consent; he is forcibly restrained while a normal segment of his body is removed; the parental consent is of quasi-legality since the part removed is a healthy, non-diseased appendage; there are no legitimate surgical-medical indications for the operation; the patient and the part operated upon are subject to a host of possible complications, including death; the genitalia are now irrevocably diminished in appearance, function and sensitivity.

Most Americans have never seen nor experienced a sexually functioning foreskin. The thoughtless, wanton amputation of an exceedingly valuable segment of male genital anatomy never ceases to amaze me. It has always been difficult for me to understand why anyone would wish to subtract one iota from genital pleasure.

The title of this chapter may be a bit inflammatory. I meant it to be. The masquerade that the circumcised penis is an alternate penile form, as good as, or possibly better than the normal structure, must end. Let us be honest! What beats the normal? How can one improve upon that which is normal? I want the reader of this book to be uncomfortable and possibly a bit angry. I want to move the American parent and male off their false base of complacent acceptance of the desensitizing, defunctionalizing operation of circumcision. We cannot change that which is past. But let us not continue to repeat the same mistake with each generation of American males out of a false, irrational, emotional, biased obstinacy.

I want this book to pique and entice, so that it is read thoughtfully from cover to cover. The reader will then be in a position to make a valid judgment of the subject.

I make no apologies, and I admit my bias for championing that which is normal.

The crowning blow to my forbearance of "routine circumcision" was the day that I examined a mixed ethnic bag of high school football players in the local Catholic high school, similar to the school that I had attended. Everyone was circumcised! I thought back to my own school days when it was still fashionable to sport a normal penis. Somehow I didn't feel that all this new-fangled surgical tailoring of penises was contributing much to medical progress. And I knew that if I had asked the student, the parent, or the physician who had performed the circumcision why it was done, none of them could give me a sound reason for the performance of the operation.

So, in my frustration, I took Bismarck's sage advice: "Righteous indignation is no substitute for a good course of action." I could no longer contain my anger at this stupid mutilation of the American male's genitals. This essay then is my "good course of action."

2. Circumcision Is Really Foreskin Amputation, and Is Abusive

The saga of man's inhumanity to man pre-dates recorded history. What follows in this book is an account of my growing awareness of one facet of this inhumanity: the persistent, compulsive need of one human being to alter the genitals of another human being. Specifically, the current practice in the United States of routine circumcision of newborn males.

You must understand something of my background. I am a first generation American. My mother was from Central Europe. Both my parents spoke fluent English, German, and "Pennsylvania Dutch." My parochial schoolmates predominantly were first generation Americans with a smattering of actual immigrants. Their families spoke German in their homes. Two of our Sunday masses were in German. One of our priests was a former chaplain in the German army. My hometown was Pennsylvania Dutch. My next-door neighbor, constant playmate, and best friend was a Jew. I am an anonymous Christian; I believe in God. I mention all these things to give you a feeling for my predisposition.

To return to my subject: none of my brothers, cousins, older relatives, nor classmates were circumcised. I never saw a circumcised penis in my early youth. Eventually I saw my neighbor's.

The difference in male genital anatomy became apparent to me over a period of years and in varying ways.

As Catholics, my family went to Sunday mass and also went to mass on Holy Days. One such Holy Day, "The Feast of the Circumcision," occurred on January 1st. (Since my mother's death the name has been changed to "Mary, Mother of God.") My mother was a devout woman but she always attended mass on this particular Holy Day under protest. She was vocal in her anger: One did not create and celebrate a church Holy Day to commemorate an act as obscene as circumcision. There was no logic in sanctifying the destruction of a normal structure that God had just created. My mother's opinion carried a lot of weight with me. A seed of doubt about this "circumcision bit" was sown in my mind. Over the years I have never found a valid counter-argument to refute my mother's humane, simple logic.

In my growing awareness of sex, I recall my mother's recounting the events of the day that my neighbor's younger brother was circumcised. Two bearded men came to our neighbor's home and circumcised the baby. My mother was angry that these men hurt the baby, and she also was concerned that the child might develop an infection. (There were no antibiotics then.) She scolded that the event was a cruel mutilation inflicted upon a helpless child's genitals.

One of my older sisters married and eventually had a baby boy, my parent's first grandchild. My sister's "progressive doctor" circumcised the child without permission, and following the operation, my nephew's penis bled profusely from a frenular artery hemorrhage. We thought the baby was going to die. My sister was beside herself with grief, as were my parents and our entire family. My nephew did not die but his permanently deformed urethral meatus and frenulum bear witness to his brief encounter with his "progressive" doctor.

I mulled over this business of circumcision. I had discovered my foreskin, and I could not fathom why anyone would want to alter or remove this neat gadget.

In discussions with my buddies, as I progressed in school, many fascinating sexual tidbits came to light. I was an Altar Boy and our mild rivals were the Choir Boys. I learned about the Vatican Choir Boys and the "boy sopranos"—"the castrati" and what was done to them to obtain more mileage from their soprano voices—I immediately knew there was one choir that I would not care to join.

And eventually in school, we studied about the Crusades. From some

---

- *What follows in this book is an account of my growing awareness of one facet of this inhumanity: the persistent, compulsive need of a human being to alter the genitals of another human being.*

- *I had discovered my foreskin, and I could not fathom why anyone would want to alter or remove this neat gadget.*

- *I learned about the Vatican Choir Boys and the "boy sopranos"—"the castrati" and what was done to them to obtain more mileage from their soprano voices.*

- *The eunuchs not only lost their testicles, but also their penises.*

2. (continued)
Circumcision Is Really Foreskin Amputation, and Is Abusive

- *This operation, still practiced today in large areas of Africa and the Islamic world, guaranteed obliteration of female genital sensation, and created a mechanical barrier to intercourse. The Muslims also practice circumcision of the male.*

- *An analogous situation exists today in the United States where the circumcised penis is accepted as the norm.*

- *Today, in most African and in many Islamic countries, mutilation of the female genitals is widespread. Egypt, Sudan, and adjacent areas still practice infibulation (i.e. excision of the clitoris and varying segments of the vulvar lips.)*

- *Surprisingly, or not surprisingly, this female genital mutilation is performed by women, who themselves have been genitally mutilated.*

unauthorized clandestine source I found out about the harems. This opened a Pandora's box of lascivious daydreams. I had all sorts of impure thoughts. It was marvelous!

Then I heard about the guardians of the harems, the eunuchs. Those boys had to pay a heavy price for their voyeurism. The Vatican-Boy-Soprano Operation was trivial, by comparison. The eunuchs not only lost their testicles, but also their penises. I was horrified. Things were getting rough!

The matter of chastity belts came to light. I didn't know then that the chastity belt was a rather improbable, seldom-used, fanciful contrivance but that the idea stemmed from what the Crusaders had learned in the Islamic countries—the practice of female infibulation: the removal of the clitoris and lesser vulvar lips, with a joining together of the raw amputated vulvar remnants. This operation, still practiced today in large areas of Africa and the Islamic world, guaranteed obliteration of female genital sensation, and created a mechanical barrier to intercourse.

The Muslims also practice circumcision of the male. So everyone in this harem scenario had some surgical, genital tailoring. The guards—the Eunuchs—had their external genitals removed completely; the women had their genitals mutilated and obtunded; and the few privileged men having access to this madhouse had their penises altered as well. Why was everyone being so nasty? I became thoroughly disenchanted with the harem and the Thousand and One Nights nonsense. The harems were not places of sexual pleasure and fantasy; they were warrens of sadistic, psychotic ugliness.

Later I learned about the Chinese courts and their techniques of creating eunuchs: the victim was held down, his scrotum and penis were grasped and twisted tightly, and then the entire external genitalia was severed flush with the perineum. A plug was inserted into the urethral stump in an effort to maintain the identity of the urethra, a clumsy attempt was made to control the bleeding, and then there was a period of waiting to see whether the eunuch would die of hemorrhage, infection or urinary complications.

From the Tarzan movies, the Travelogues, the *National Geographic*, etc., I became apprised of other, less violent forms of mutilation: Ubangis with deformed lips and noses, natives with elongated heads and necks, skin scarification with resultant keloid patterns, and so forth. I learned too of the Chinese women having their feet bound, ostensibly to enhance their beauty. It seemed incongruous that the normal feet would be perceived as ugly and the abnormally deformed feet would be viewed as beautiful. An analogous situation exists today in the United States where the circumcised penis is accepted, by most, as the norm.

Today, in most African and in many Islamic countries, mutilation of the female genitals is widespread.[1] Egypt, Sudan, and adjacent areas still practice infibulation (i.e. excision of the clitoris and varying segments of the vulvar lips.) In more primitive areas of Africa, the clitoris, a convex structure with a vestigial connotation of maleness, is destroyed by burning it with a hot object. Male circumcision, which is also widespread in Africa and the Islamic nations, does not have as horrible sequelae as does this sadistic mutilation of the female. Surprisingly, or not surprisingly, this female genital mutilation is performed by women, who themselves have been genitally mutilated.

Penile Structures[2]

External penile structures can be more easily understood by first describing a circumcised penis. Its outward appearance is that of a cylinder, rounded at the end. Four parts are visible, namely: the shaft, which makes up the major length of the organ; the glans or rounded head at the end; the sulcus, or groove, which separates the glans from the shaft; and the meatus, or opening at the tip of the glans, which permits passage of urine and semen (see Figure 1).

A normal, intact penis has each of the four parts mentioned above plus a foreskin. The foreskin, or prepuce, can be visualized as cone-shaped with the base of the cone encircling the penile shaft, close to the groove. The foreskin is also attached to the underside of the glans at a ridge called the frenulum (also called the frenum). Usually, the foreskin covers the glans completely, although in some cases it may only cover it partly or it may extend beyond it, as there are variations from person to person. Though the foreskin is cone-shaped, the tip is not pointed but is instead blunt and has an opening. Because the foreskin fits snugly over the glans, which is often wider than the shaft, the foreskin appears to bulge at the widest part of the glans (see Figure 2). Thus the foreskin can be visualized as a soft, pliable, cone-shaped tissue, which is open at the end to permit the passage of urine and semen from the meatus. The opening is expandable in order to allow for the protrusion of the glans in erection, for washing the glans, and for urination after infancy.

Actually, the foreskin is composed of two distinct layers of tissue, almost like a lined sleeve. The inner layer starts from the foreskin opening at the tip, where it is joined to the outer foreskin layer, and continues under the outer layer to cover the glans (see Figure 3). The inner layer is attached to the shaft near the groove, or sulcus, as well as to the underside of the glans at the frenum.

Unlike the inner layer, the outer layer of the foreskin is simply an extension of the external skin of the penile shaft, which continues over the glans until it joins the inner layer at the opening at the tip of the foreskin. The outer layer does not come into direct contact with the glans.

The two foreskin layers are different in structure and function. The texture of the outer layer is identical to the rest of the penile shaft skin and, as with all penile skin, it is erotogenic. The texture of the foreskin inner lining is that of a mucous membrane and it is kept moist by the secretion of smegma, which its cells produce. The inner layer also contains specialized nerve cells which make it one of the more erotogenic of all male body tissues. (The inner lining of the clitoral foreskin is similarly endowed.)

When an intact penis is flaccid (not erect), the entire organ is covered with a continuum of skin from the base (at the abdomen) to the meatus. In a circumcised penis, the external skin ends near the groove, which is usually exposed, as are the glans and the meatus.

Infant Circumcision Procedure

Modern medical circumcision means amputation of both layers of the foreskin. This operation is performed on baby boys in their first few days after birth.

Presurgical Preparations

1. First, the baby is strapped to a restraint board to prevent thrashing during the procedure. Most modern boards hold the arms and legs with Velcro straps. The arms are strapped by the baby's side near his hips, and his legs are held down with straps around the thighs in a slightly separated position.

2. The genital area of the baby is cleaned with an antiseptic scrub, and then the baby's body is draped, totally covered with a sterile cloth except for a small hole through which the penis protrudes.

3. The baby may be given an injection of local anesthetic directly into his penis, although this is relatively uncommon.

There are two popular methods of infant circumcision—the Gomco technique (Figure 4) and the Plastibell technique (Figure 5). Following is a brief description of each. Note the cautions in the descriptions. These emphasize that complications can and do occur. Circumcision is not trivial surgery.

2. *(continued)*
Circumcision Is Really Foreskin Amputation, and Is Abusive

2. *(continued)*
Circumcision Is Really Foreskin Amputation, and Is Abusive

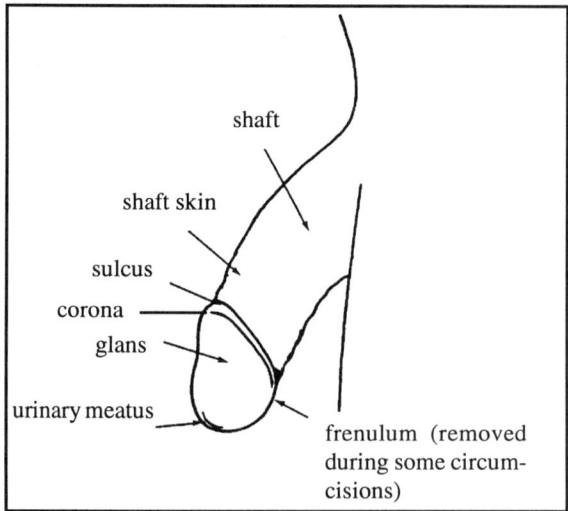

Figure 1. Flaccid circumcised adult penis

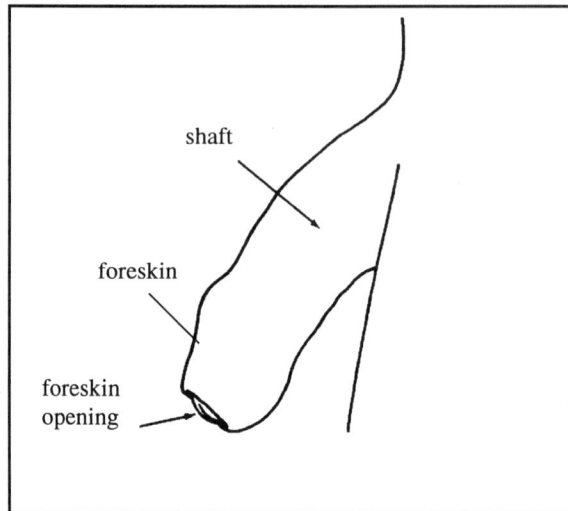

Figure 2. Flaccid normal intact adult penis

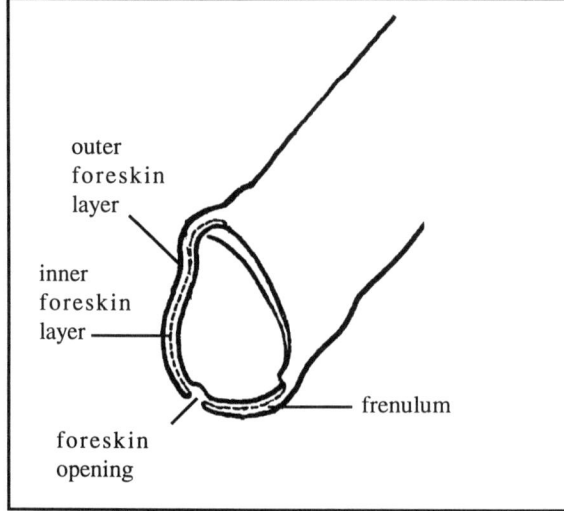

Figure 3. Hidden view showing foreskin layers of flaccid normal intact adult penis

2. *(continued)* Circumcision Is Really Foreskin Amputation, and Is Abusive

The Gomco Technique[3]

1. Stretch the preputial opening.
2. Break preputial adhesions* so that the foreskin is completely retractile (A).
3. Retract the foreskin until you can see the corona. Check the glans for any hidden adhesions*. If the entire preputial space is not free, you stand a good chance of pinching the glans on the bell or clamp, or of leaving adhesions behind.
4. Apply a small amount of lubricant such as K-Y jelly to the glans so that it won't stick to the inside of the bell.
5. Apply the bell-shaped plunger over the glans. The bell should fit easily over the glans so that it covers the corona. Too small a bell may injure the glans and fail to protect the corona. If stretching the preputial opening does not allow the bell to be inserted in the preputial space and entirely cover the glans, a dorsal slit may be necessary. (B)
6. Pull the prepuce up over the bell. The foreskin should not be stretched or pulled too snugly over the bell. If it's pulled up too tightly, it's possible to remove too much shaft skin or to pull the urethra up so you get a tangential cut through the urethra as well as the skin. (C)
7. Judge the amount of the shaft skin left below the corona; the skin should be relaxed and supple.
8. After you're sure of the dimensions, apply the plate of the clamp at the level of the corona. (D)
9. With everything in proper alignment, tighten the clamp. This squeezes the prepuce between the bell and the clamp to make it blood-free. Be sure the weight of the clamp doesn't distort the anatomy so there isn't the proper amount of skin in the clamp.
10. Make a circumferential incision with a cold knife, not an electrosurgical instrument. (E)
11. Leave the clamp in place at least five minutes to allow clotting and coaptation to occur.
12. Remove the clamp and apply antiseptic ointment (Betadine) to the crush line. Apply a light dressing or loin cloth arrangement to keep the ointment from rubbing off.
13. If you remove the clamp prematurely, the crushed edges may separate and bleeding will occur. When this occurs, suture the mucocutaneous margin, being careful to avoid deep, sutures that might penetrate the urethra. If the whole edge separates, treat as a freehand circumcision, placing quadrant sutures and sewing between them with fine stitches.
14. Have the baby watched overnight for any sign of bleeding.
15. If late separation occurs, it's best to keep the wound clean and let it heal secondarily rather than to try to suture it and risk development of stricture or fistula. Skin of this area tends to re-epithelialize rapidly.

*A tragic misnomer, since the foreskin is almost always naturally attached to the glans at birth.

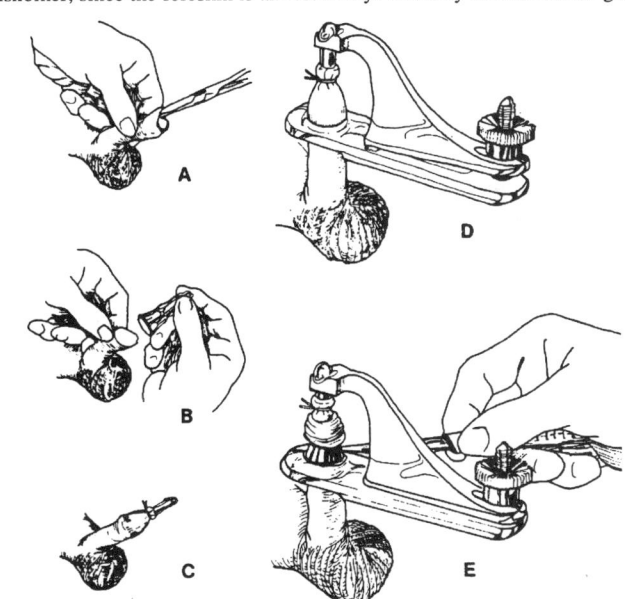

Figure 4. The Gomco technique of circumcision

2. (continued)
Circumcision Is Really Foreskin Amputation, and Is Abusive

The Plastibell Technique[3]

1. Stretch the preputial opening.
2. Break preputial adhesions* with a probe or closed forceps.
3. Make a small dorsal slit of 0.5 to 1.0 cm in the prepuce. Keep the initial slit short; it can always be extended. To minimize bleeding, previously crush the line of incision with artery forceps for one minute. Take particular care not to place forceps or scissors in the urethra meatus; before cutting or crushing, lift the prepuce away from the glans and visualize the meatus. (A,B)
4. Separate the edges of the slit with a pair of artery forceps to reveal the glans. If necessary, extend the cut to expose the coronal sulcus. (C)
5. Free any remaining adhesions* and lay the prepuce back (inside out) to expose the entire glans.
6. Slip the Plastibell of appropriate size over the glans as far as the coronal sulcus. It should slip over the glans easily; too small a bell may injure the glans.
7. Place the prepuce over the bell to hold it in place. (D)
8. Tie the ligature as tightly as possible around the prepuce on the ridge of the bell; oozing will occur if the ligature is loose.
9. After one to two minutes to allow for crush, trim off the prepuce at the distal edge of the ligature, using a knife or scissors. Trim as much tissue as possible to reduce the amount of necrotic tissue and possibility of infection. (E)
10. Snap off the handle of the bell, leaving the bell and ligature in place. You should be able to see an unobstructed urethral meatus. (F)
11. No dressing is necessary; the baby may be bathed normally; the rim of tissue under and distal to the ligature will become necrotic (dead) and will separate with the bell in 5 to 10 days.
12. Occasionally, edema will trap the plastic ring on the shaft of the penis. In this case, it's usually necessary to cut off the ring, using a guide and ring cutter, although application of ice will sometimes reduce edema enough to remove the ring.

*A tragic misnomer, since the foreskin is almost always naturally attached to the glans at birth.

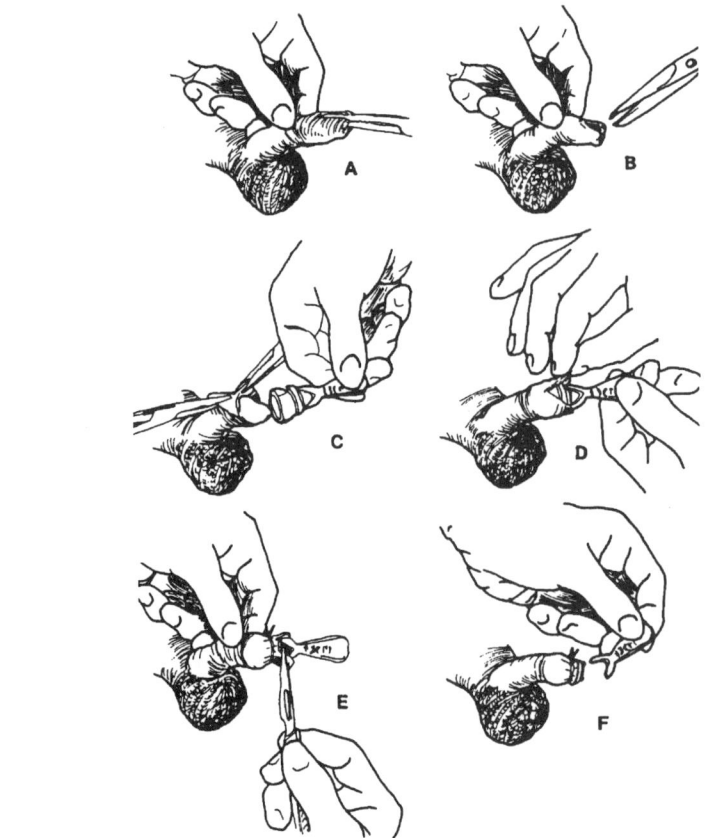

Figure 5. The Plastibell technique of circumcision

3. Circumcision Is Very Painful and Traumatizing—A Terrible Way to Welcome Your Newborn Baby Boy

In the course of every circumcision, all babies scream, tremble, and/or cry. Many hold their breath or vomit. Some cry for hours afterward, and remain irritable for days. Studies have been done on how this stress impacts upon adrenal cortical function, upon decreased arterial oxygen perfusion in response to pain, and disturbance of sleep-awake states. Every impartial observer must agree that circumcision performed upon an unanesthetized infant is an exceedingly stressful ordeal. Every parent should witness this "benign" operation.

The great human and humane transgression is that we have taken a helpless, dependent infant and needlessly subjected him to pain.

Could one repair an inguinal hernia in a newborn infant without benefit of *any* anesthesia on the presumption that the newborn's perception of pain is not sufficiently developed so as to warrant an anesthetic?

In our area recently, the parents of a small child were convicted of child abuse when they "disciplined" their small child by burning the skin with a heated teaspoon. Is such an action any more cruel than removing an intact, sensitive, normal foreskin from a penis without anesthesia? What constitutes child abuse?

Another paradox exists: Great strides have been made in obstetrics. We are aware that the child in the course of delivery must be well oxygenated, not sedated, and gently cared for. Hopefully, the infant is accepted with love. Then, within a day or two after delivery, if the infant is a male, he is strapped to a restraining board, subjected to bright lights and cold instruments, and without benefit of anesthesia* his foreskin is amputated. There is something terribly bizarre, incongruous and irrational about this course of action.

And even if local anesthesia were used, the anesthetic effect lasts but an hour or two. Then the pain at the amputation site returns. Now it is impossible to avoid contact between the unprotected, raw, reddened, exquisitely sensitive glans penis and feces or urine-soaked diapers. Even holding the infant to comfort him inflicts pain. It takes about ten to fourteen days until the amputation site heals and the pain subsides. But now glans contact with feces, urine, and diapers is unavoidable until the child is "potty-trained" since the normal protective sleeve of the foreskin is gone forever.

- *A helpless, dependent infant is subjected needlessly to pain!*

- *Would one repair an inguinal hernia in a neonatal infant without anesthesia?*

- *According to current ethical guidelines, surgical procedures cannot be performed on **research animals** without using anesthesia. But historically, neonatal circumcision has been done **without** anesthesia.*

- *"Changes in heart rate, respiratory rate, transcutaneous pO2, adrenal cortical hormone secretion, sleep patterns, and behavioral patterns have been shown to be altered during and/or following circumcision of the full-term neonate. Indeed, circumcision has been recommended as a model for studying pain in the neonate, and its effects are suggested to be long-lasting."*

    Suzanne Dixon, M.D.

Victims' Voices...

"I didn't know what circumcision was when I consented to have my three sons circumcised. My doctor had told me the surgery was a necessary health measure, that it didn't hurt, and that it only took a moment to perform...like cutting the umbilical cord, I thought. I certainly wasn't prepared when, in nursing school several years later, I saw the surgery for the first time.

We students filed into the newborn nursery to find a baby strapped spread-eagle to a plastic board on a counter top across the room. He was struggling against his restraints—tugging, whimpering, and then crying helplessly. No one was tending the infant, but when I asked my instructor if I could comfort him she said "Wait till the doctor gets here." I wondered how a teacher of the healing arts could watch someone suffer and not offer assistance. I wondered about the doctor's power which could intimidate others from following protective instincts. When he did arrive, I immediately asked the doctor if I could help the baby. He told me to put my finger into the baby's mouth; I did, and the baby sucked. I stroked his little head and spoke softly to him. He began to relax and was momentarily quiet.

The silence was soon broken by a piercing scream—the baby's reaction to having his foreskin pinched and crushed as the doctor

---

*In newborns, anesthesia creates additional risks and potential complications.

3. (continued)
Circumcision Is Very Painful and Traumatizing—A Terrible Way to Welcome Your Newborn Baby Boy

- *... Studies recently have demonstrated that infants do indeed experience pain.*

- *"Anyone who has been present when a clamp was placed on a newborn's foreskin can never again doubt that the procedure hurts. An infant who's just gone through the stress of birth should emerge into a world that's loving and tender. Why should we attack his most precious possession? There is an increasing body of evidence that neonates, including those born preterm, demonstrate physiologic responses to surgical procedures that are similar to those demonstrated by adults."*

  Loraine Stern, M.D.

- *"The rule of thumb that I typically use is that anything that hurts an adult will hurt a child."*

  Neil L. Schechter, M.D.

Victims' Voices (continued)...

attached the clamp to his penis. The shriek intensified when the doctor inserted an instrument between the foreskin and the glans (head of the penis), tearing the two structures apart. (They are normally attached to each other during infancy so the foreskin can protect the sensitive glans from urine and feces.) The baby started shaking his head back and forth—the only part of his body free to move—as the doctor used another clamp to crush the foreskin lengthwise, which he then cut. This made the opening of the foreskin large enough to insert a circumcision instrument, the device used to protect the glans from being severed during the surgery.

The baby began to gasp and choke, breathless from his shrill continuous screams. How could anyone say circumcision is painless when the suffering is so obvious? My bottom lip began to quiver, tears filled my eyes and spilled over. I found my own sobs difficult to contain. How much longer could this go on?

During the next stage of the surgery, the doctor crushed the foreskin against the circumcision instrument and then, finally, amputated it. The baby was limp, exhausted, spent.

I had not been prepared, nothing could have prepared me, for this experience. To see a part of this baby's penis being cut off—without an anesthetic—was devastating. But even more shocking was the doctor's comment, barely audible several octaves below the piercing screams of the baby, "There's no medical reason for doing this." I couldn't believe my ears, my knees became weak, and I felt sick to my stomach. I couldn't believe that medical professionals, dedicated to helping and healing, could inflict such pain and anguish on innocent babies unnecessarily.

What had I allowed my own babies to endure and why?"

Marilyn Milos, R.N.

"As an American middle-class woman, I had always thought penises were supposed to look a certain way with the exposed, rounded head at the end. It had never occurred to me that anything was changed or cut off to make it look that way... I gave birth to our first child, a son...When the baby and I came home and I first began changing his diapers, I found that he too had a penis in the style and shape to which I was culturally accustomed, with the rounded glans exposed. The end of the baby's penis was bright red for a few days, but soon healed. The baby screamed every time his diaper was changed. Being a naive new mother, I had no idea why diaper changing upset him so much—perhaps all babies did that...

Two and a half years later, in 1974, our second son was born in another hospital... I was more aware of the baby's undergoing circumcision... Although I expected that the procedure would be painful for the baby, it never occurred to me not to have it done. Again this baby had a penis in the style which seemed "normal" to me. The new baby's penis healed within a few days and I forgot about it.

Two years later... I again became pregnant... We made the unconventional and daring decision... [to] give birth at home... The idea occurred to me that if our new baby was a boy, perhaps he should not be circumcised. However, I knew practically nothing about it. None of our doctors ever gave us any information about the operation—pros, cons, why, or how it was done... my awareness of circumcision consisted of nothing more than a basic concept of how penises were "supposed" to look and a vague idea that it was somehow supposed to be cleaner [and the author was a childbirth educator!]... Our third little son came into the world in the peace and comfort of our home... During the next few days our new son nursed contentedly, slept peacefully, and rarely cried. He had a peacefulness and serenity that I had never known with my first babies... What incomprehensible force brought me from the beautiful, untraumatized birth at home to a strange doctor's office one week later—sitting there frightened and reluctant, holding my sleeping, peaceful, trusting newborn infant? "He shouldn't be different from his brothers or father." "I'm afraid he'll have problems." "Our relatives would object if we didn't have it done." All these thoughts went through my head, while all the while I wanted so much to protect my baby from any harm. My husband and I found ourselves relinquishing our baby and leaving the building. When we returned about 15 minutes later, the office was filled with our baby's screams. I found our precious baby on the doctor's operating table with a penis that was cut, raw, and bright red! I remember his brothers' penises looking that way, but while they, to me, seemed to be born that way, this baby had definitely been injured, damaged, and traumatized!... I immediately held and nursed him, trying to relieve his pitiful screams... I felt like I had brought home a different baby. His tense, agonized little body reminded me of the way his brothers had been as newborns... The trauma and torture that was inflicted upon this tiny, helpless little being was to come back and haunt me again and again."

Rosemary Romberg

Much could be written on this topic, but often people say it best. Listen to the pain and anguish in the voices of the parents of circumcised infants, and in the voices of circumcised men, both victims of circumcision. The people included here are but a few of the thousands who have found the courage to speak out.

4. Circumcision Produces Psychological and Emotional Pain and Anguish to Sons and Parents

Victims' Voices . . .

"I can still remember his chilling screams! How could I have ever let them do that to my poor defenseless child? Every mother tries to do her best for her child, and I thought I was doing the best thing. If I had thought more about it I would have realized it (the foreskin) was there for a reason."

Betty, Dallas

"My husband held the baby to the table while the doctor performed the operation. I found the screams unbearable and retreated to a chair in the waiting room. The doctor told my husband that at that age a baby's penis isn't really that sensitive and he was screaming out of fright and not pain....There is still a scar. We realize now that we made the wrong decision and our reasoning was ridiculous. Any other male children born to us will not be circumcised."

Maggie & David, Kentucky

"They strapped him down which I hated. We massaged his head, stroked him, and talked to him the whole time....My husband said it was the most awful thing he'd ever seen or done.

Paula & Richard, Michigan

"I stood outside the door while they were doing it to him and listened to him scream and cry. That's the first time I really began to wonder what the hell I had let them do to my baby! Since then I have asked myself that a million times."

Bill, California

"After about 40 minutes the doctor came out and explained to us that there was one spot that would not stop bleeding. I don't think we were aware that there could be complications. There was no doubt in our minds that this was wrong, knowing that it wasn't necessary in the first place. It must have been torture for him....(later) He constantly cried and sniffled...this went on all day. I held Gabriel the whole day. I couldn't move him. I felt horrible! I felt like I had just killed him! I can't explain the guilt that I felt. I was angry. I hurt all over for my baby."

Betty, Oregon

"Something terrible had happened that could never be redeemed. It was like the fall from the Garden of Eden. We had this beautiful baby boy and 7 beautiful days and this beautiful rhythm starting and it was like something snatched the essence of what was ever there and damaged it!"

Marge & Frank, New York

"When I was born, I had the grave misfortune to be delivered by a doctor who convinced my mother to agree to my being circumcised. Since that day I have cursed all and sundry for the unwarranted and criminal mutilation of my penis. Perhaps I have overreacted but the loss of my foreskin has developed into a major psychological problem to such extent that I have had to undergo prolonged psychoanalysis, but the fixation is so firmly implanted in my mind that no amount of treatment has had any effect whatsoever. I would sell my soul to the Devil ten times over if I could get my foreskin back again. I have two sons who sport two magnificent long, loose foreskins, the sight of which turns me green with envy. I had to defend their foreskins and their right to retain them, almost with violence, such is the circumcision mania among doctors. God made men's penises with foreskins because they are supposed to have one and I want mine back. I've developed an abso-

- *"If there is one thing about his birth that I could take back, circumcision would be it."*

Concerned mother

4. (continued)
Circumcision Produces Psychological and Emotional Pain and Anguish to Sons and Parents

Victims' Voices (continued)...

lute fixation in regard to foreskins in general, and my lack of one in particular, so please forgive me."

M.G., Father of two intact sons

"When we (men) discuss circumcision, and the pros of not being cut, no one listens, not even doctors. I am one of millions of men who does not like the fact that I am circumcised. I never have liked it, and wish I had been able as a baby to sit up and scream at the doctor to `take your hands off, that's mine.' I am still envious of men who I see who are intact. I have always exercised in a local Y or gym and have seen thousands of boys and men in the showers over the years. The American male's penis is a ruined penis. In most cases, too much skin has been removed, thus during erection there is no sheath movement of the outer skin. Penis `function' is then nonexistent. Some friends have shown me that their careless circumcision resulted in up to half of the glans being removed. `Thanks a lot doctors,' we appreciate what you've done for us."

S.B., 47, Atlanta

"At age 70, I will always remember the pain of my circumcision, at age 7, while under ether for a tonsillectomy. How I wish I still had my foreskin. I didn't know what had happened at the time. It's sad when we have no voice in a decision."

R.D., Wisconsin

"I am a male 24 years old. This is a personal and emotional subject for me, and I am having much difficulty in writing this. I am so angry and upset and depressed that I've been circumcised. How can someone think that they know so much that they can decide to surgically modify/mutilate my sexual organs without even consulting me? I remember (age under 8) being in the tub bathing. I had noticed a brown ring of tissue around my penis and (my mother was in the bathroom at the time) asked my mother what it was. She replied, `That's where you were circumcised.' I asked why. She replied, `To keep it clean.' I thought it was a poor reason. I have since my early teens wished to have my foreskin reconstructed. At that time, I had not heard of it ever being done, but I had heard of sex change operations and figured, by comparison, that foreskin reconstruction would be a piece of cake. When my first serious girlfriend offered to perform fellatio on me I happily agreed. However, when it happened, I felt practically nothing; I thanked her and told her it was wonderful—a lie. I was disappointed, but I said to myself, `It was the first time. Maybe I was nervous. And it was in the back of my car—not the ideal place for an orgasm.' A few months later, at the age of 17, I lost my virginity to her; it too was disappointing. I could not feel anything and did not have an orgasm. Of the 30 to 40 times I had intercourse with her I achieved orgasm/ejaculation only 4 or 5 times. I tried it both with and without a condom. It felt slightly better without, but not enough to matter, and I knew it wasn't a good idea. Now I am with the most wonderful woman in the world. I'm deeply in love with her. She is sexy, has some erotic `naughty nighties,' and my sex life with her has been much better than the others. At first it wasn't, but she gave me time, and now my frequency of orgasm is up to about 1 in 4. This is great compared to before, but I still feel like I'm missing something. My hypothesis is that my lack of sensitivity is due to not only the physiological changes circumcision causes, but mentally as well."

C.A., Sacramento

"The scars of circumcision are not only on the infant. A neighbor commented recently that she didn't like `the circumcision thing' and went on to recall that she had heard her new son crying continuously for two days after he was circumcised. He was in a nursery down the hall from her hospital room, but through two sleepless nights, she could recognize his voice among all the others. She was 89 when she told the story, her son 55. That's a long time to carry feelings of guilt and inadequacy. What a pall to cast over what should be a pinnacle of joy!"

M.J., Illinois

5. Circumcision Creates Unnecessary Surgical Risks and Complications

Many events propelled me into this crusade against routine male circumcision. For many years I performed physical examinations in the elementary and high schools. This encompassed examinations of children in kindergarten, seventh, and eleventh grades, as well as members of the various athletic teams associated with the schools. In examining the boys, I was struck by two things: the ubiquitousness of circumcisions in the United States, and the inordinately large number of badly performed circumcisions with resultant deformed penises.

Anyone who has conducted similar examinations of males, as well as anyone who has been in the Armed Forces or who has frequented gyms and public showers, has observed these same things. One sees circumcised penises that incline to the right or left; those that have adhesions of the circumcised skin edges to the corona with varying thicknesses of skin bridging; glans whose tips are truncated by a too closely placed cut, etc. If one looks a bit more closely at the urethral meatus (urinary openings), many of the openings are rounded, narrowed, and often pinpoint, instead of possessing the dumbbell-like slit of the normal penis. This meatal narrowing occurs *only* in those circumcised and has an incidence of about one-third in all those who are circumcised.

The practice of operating upon a normal structure—the foreskin—must produce consternation in many physicians, especially when they have monitored the results, and have discovered that the operation is not without its immediate and future complications.

Look at this finding from the Council of Scientific Affairs of the American Medical Association in 1987: "Both the Gomco clamp and the Plastibell instruments are associated with complications of pain and hemorrhage (1% of cases) and infection (0.4%). The complication rate ranges from 0.6% in one study to a high of 55% in another study. Meatal ulceration may occur in 8% to 31% of cases. Surgical complications, e.g., wound dehiscence, bridging of skin between penile shaft and glans, and denuding of the penile shaft are relatively common. Urinary retention, chordee, cysts, lymphedema, necrosis, hypospadias and fistulas also may occur."

In the United States the possibility of a serious complication as a result of an infant circumcision is estimated, by a doctor who favors circumcision, to be one in every 500 operations. (Gee WF, Ansell JS. Neonatal Circumcision—a ten year overview. Pediatrics 58:824, 1976) Therefore, the statistical probability of a serious surgical complication being caused by circumcision is 200 times higher than the likelihood of getting cancer of the penis.[4]

In Britain in 1946, one child in 6,000 under the age of 5 died as a result of circumcision complications.[5] If one applies this statistical probability to the United States, there would be hundreds of deaths per year. In investigating deaths related to circumcision in the United States, one must realize that the litigious malpractice milieu existing here makes accurate reporting of such deaths very suspect.

It would take great courage and honesty on the part of a United States physician to report a death attributable to circumcision, when that physician knows that the procedure has been deemed unnecessary by the American pediatric and obstetrical societies, and that he may be sued for malpractice.

This operation of circumcision seems to be an odd bird, being neither fish nor fowl. In the minds of many it is really not an operation at all.

Third party insurance carriers, the American Medical Association, and the American College of Surgeons do not consider it, nor mention it, as amongst the ten or twelve most commonly performed operations in the United States. And yet it is the most frequently performed operation. Insurance carriers do not request a "second opinion" prior to its performance.

- *There is an inordinately large number of badly performed circumcisions with resultant deformed penises.*

- *In the United States, the statistical probability of a serious medical complication being caused by circumcision is much higher than the likelihood of getting cancer of the penis.*

- *Accurate reporting of deaths attributed to circumcision is very suspect.*

- *"Such problems (i.e. urethral meatal narrowing) virtually never occur in uncircumcised penises. The foreskin protects the glans throughout life."*
  American Academy of Pediatrics

- *The Food and Drug Administration (FDA) received 105 reports of injuries involving circumcision clamps between July 1996 and January 2000. These included lacerations, hemorrhage, penile amputation and urethral damage.*

5. (continued)
Circumcision Creates Unnecessary Surgical Risks and Complications

- *In no other operation does the layman make the exclusive decision to operate.*

- *The removal of 100% normal foreskins, year after year, never merits one word of comment nor censure from any Tissue Committee.*

- *In assessing any complication, one must remember that one started with a normal penis.*

- *Fatal hemorrhage can occur following neonatal circumcision.*

- *Meatal ulceration occurs only in the circumcised.*

- *The normal urinary stream in the male is a spiraling ribbon. The urinary stream in meatal stenosis is needle-like, prolonged, and frequently associated with discomfort.*

The holistic medical groups, the La Leche League, and various organizations concerned with maternal-child bonding apparently do not think it odd to advocate the delivery of the child with warmth and gentleness, lowered lights, and subdued noise—as counseled by Doctor LeBoyer—and then in the next day or so subjecting that infant to the harsh realities of a painful operation without anesthesia.

Actually few people take neonatal circumcision seriously. Tissue Committees, that exist in every accredited hospital and pass judgment upon whether an operation is justified, give no thought to the matter. If the number of normal appendices, gall bladders, uteri, etc. removed by any surgeon exceeds an acceptable average, that surgeon would be censored or even dismissed from the hospital staff. It is utterly beyond imagination for a surgeon to consistently remove normal appendices, gall bladders, etc. 100% of the time, and not have the matter discussed and acted upon by the Tissue Committee. But the removal of 100% normal foreskins, year after year, never merits one word of comment or censure by any Tissue Committee. One might merely joke about the little raisin-like, shriveled, formalin-soaked foreskin in the specimen bottle.

Complications of Circumcision

The general categories of complications are those of: blood loss, infection, and mechanical or structural abnormalities. Here are the specifics:

Hemorrhage: Bleeding from the frenular artery can be brisk, and if undetected for only a moderately short time, can be fatal. A three kilogram infant (6.6 pounds) has a total blood volume of roughly eight ounces—a drinking glass capacity. It is estimated that serious hemorrhage occurs in at least 2% of infants. Fatal hemorrhage does occur. Hemorrhagic shock is more common. Venous bleeding is seldom a problem.

Urinary Retention: This can be secondary to swelling from the trauma of the operation, from surgical dressings, from pain associated with attempts at urination, or from mechanical devices, specifically the Plastibell device.

Laceration of Penile and Scrotal Skin: This can be of varying degree.

Excessive Penile Skin Loss: If the tip of the prepuce is drawn forward too vigorously and the circumcising bell crushing clamp is applied, almost the entire penile skin sheath can be removed. The individual now has an unending problem with penile bowing and pain at the time of erection. Skin grafting may be needed to correct the excessive skin loss. Improper placement of the circumcision bell with unequal traction of the foreskin at the time of the bell application can result in an unequal skin removal anywhere along the circumference of the circumcising cut. Thus the penis can permanently deviate or bow in any direction depending upon the amount or the location of the skin removed.

Beveling Deformities of the Glans: Any physician who has examined many penises sees this deformity from time to time. Varying amounts of the tip of the glans penis inadvertently have been shaved off through carelessness on the part of the doctor. The transected area eventually heals, leaving a scarred beveled surface. There are documented cases of the entire glans being amputated.

Hypospadias Deformity: This is produced by the inadvertent drawing of the frenular area too far forward and then after applying the crushing bell, injuring the urethra at the time the foreskin is removed with the knife. This results in a urethral opening on the undersurface of the penile shaft.

Epispadias Deformity: This occurs when one limb of the crushing clamp which is meant to engage only the undersurface of the foreskin inadvertently is passed into the urethra. When the clamp is closed, it crushes the upper portion of the urethra, the upper part of the glans penis, and the foreskin. The tragic result is a urethral opening on the top of the glans.

Retention of the Plastibell Ring: The Plastibell device and the Gomco clamp are the two most commonly used mechanical aids for circumcising infants. With the Plastibell, the bell remains on the end of the penis for about ten days before it (the bell) sloughs off. The

5. *(continued)*
Circumcision Creates Unnecessary Surgical Risks and Complications

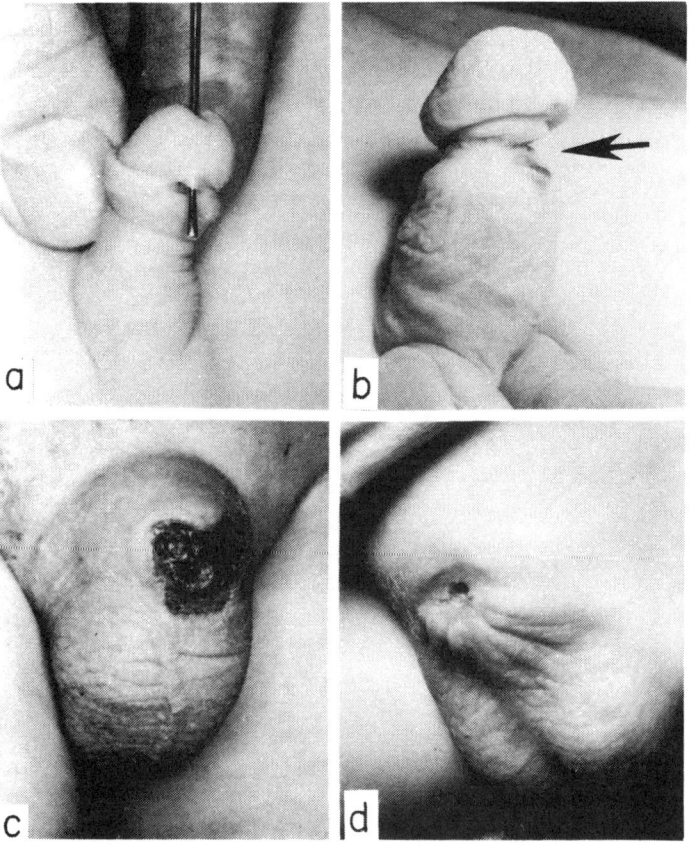

Complications of circumcision. *A*, Urethral fistula at frenulum (note probe), probably the result of incisional trauma. *B*, Three-year-old boy with an almost transected glans from circumcision at birth, but parents did not note the abnormality until age 3. Urethra had been completely transected (arrow). Repair included reanastomosing the ends of the urethra and repair of deep cleft surrounding corpora. *C*, Neonate referred immediately after Gomco clamp circumcision in which all the skin of the shaft had been amputated. This is a fairly common complication caused by pulling too much skin up into the clamp and amputating it. Fortunately sometimes there is enough of the mucosal side of the prepuce to fold back to resurface the shaft, but some require a free skin graft. *D*, Six-month-old baby was referred after loss of the entire penis from cautery used during circumcision. Evidently both corpora had thrombosed and sloughed, so no phallus remained.

Figure 6. Some circumcision complications. From the textbook *Pediatric Trauma*, edited by Robert J. Touloukian, M.D., Yale University School of Medicine (John Wiley & Sons). Used with permission.

5. (continued)
Circumcision Creates Unnecessary Surgical Risks and Complications

- *Meatal stenosis (narrowing) occurs in about one-third of all neonatal circumcisions. It takes several years to become apparent.*

- *Many physicians fall short of questioning the need for operating upon a normal structure (the foreskin).*

- *Most U.S. physicians do not know that the foreskin has important functions.*

- *If one performs an unnecessary operation upon a normal structure, one can accept nothing more than zero mortality, zero morbidity, zero complications, and zero unfavorable end results!*

- *Most Americans are too ill-informed to question physician-induced penile deformities.*

plastic device may get buried under the skin of the penile shaft. Ulceration and/or necrosis of the skin at and beyond the bell can occur. Necrosis and loss of the glans have been reported.

Chordee: This is dense scarring at the frenular area causing bowing of the penis upon erection. A corrective Z-plasty operation may be needed to remedy the deformity.

Keloid Formation: Keloids are excessively prominent scars which can occur anywhere on the body. On the end of the penis, the excessive scar can occur wherever the skin-mucous membrane has been incised, crushed, or sutured.

Lymphedema: If infection and/or surgical trauma blocks lymphatic return, the head of the penis [or glans] can become chronically swollen.

Concealed Penis: The circumcised penis retreats and becomes hidden in the fat pad of the pubic area.

Skin Bridges: This is scar tissue that forms bridges between the raw skin of the head of the penis and the shaft skin. Skin bridges are common and consist of thick areas of transected skin from the distal penile shaft, bridging the corona, and attaching to the raw glans.

Phimosis of Remaining Foreskin: This may happen if only a segment of the foreskin is removed. The remaining tip of the foreskin becomes tight and nonretractable, and despite the circumcision, the glans still cannot be seen. A re-operation may become necessary.

Preputial Cysts: Islands of skin or mucous membrane can be implanted along the line of circumcision closure. Or infection or mechanical distortion can block normal sweat or sebaceous glands. Cysts can result.

Cosmetic Problems: "Untidy" skin tags can occur at the line of circumcision.

Loss of Penis: There are several causes: infection, constricting rings (e.g. Plastibell), or use of the electrocautery device. A sex change operation has been used as one unhappy solution.

Infections: These can be localized to the genital area or remote from the area. All of the following and more have been reported in the medical literature: "scalded skin" and necrosis of the perineum, necrotizing fasciitis of the abdominal wall, localized diphtheria and tuberculosis, tetanus (especially in Third World countries), lung abscess, osteomyelitis (bone infection), meningitis, and bacteremia.

Death: this is the ultimate tragic complication.

Meatitis: Neonatal circumcision also predisposes to meatitis (inflammation of the urinary opening) which may progress to meatal stenosis (narrowing of the opening). As far back as 1921, Brenneman taught that meatal ulceration occurred only in the circumcised baby. Mackenzie observed an incidence of such ulceration following circumcision in more than 20% of infants. It now seems incontrovertible that such ulceration leads to meatal stenosis (narrowing) of varying degrees. Most of these cases cause no apparent trouble, but some do progress to pinpoint urethral openings. There is a theoretical and actual possibility that some obstruction to the urinary tract may occur.

Meatal Ulceration: Occurs when the unprotected urethra opening at the tip of the penis is abraded against dry and wet diapers, soiled with urine and feces. It is estimated that meatal ulceration occurs in 50% of all circumcised infants. Meatal ulceration does not occur in the normal infant penis.

Meatal Stricture: This is an advanced degree of meatal ulceration. With persistent or excessive ulceration, the scar tissue contracts and narrows the urethral opening. The urethral meatus loses its normal slit-like, dumbbell-shaped contour and becomes round and sometimes pinpoint. Varying degrees of urinary obstruction are theoretically possible. If the stenosis becomes too severe, a surgical meatotomy (enlarging of the meatus) may be necessary. Again, the condition is iatrogenic (doctor-produced), and is not found in the normal penis protected by a foreskin. It occurs in about one-third of all circumcised babies. Meatal stenosis usually is not apparent for several years. Ironically, often the obstetrician, the individual responsible for this condition, does not have the benefit of patient follow-up and is blithely ignorant of what he's caused.

5. *(continued)* Circumcision Creates Unnecessary Surgical Risks and Complications

Summary

Interestingly, many physicians, upon reviewing the complications of circumcision merely conclude their estimation by calling for greater skill and care in performing the procedure. They fail to question the need for operating upon a normal structure. Probably most physicians in the United States are too sexually unimaginative to know that the foreskin has important functions.

An article appearing recently in one of the popular women's magazines indicates how ignorant the average American woman is of male genital anatomy, and how accepting she is of iatrogenic (doctor-produced) genital deformities. Included in the article was the following: "A penis may be beautifully curved or elegantly straight; it may veer to the left or the right . . ."

This particular magazine is read by millions of women, and articles by so-called experts are probably accepted as the truth. The woman author undoubtedly is truthfully reporting what she has observed and read. The tragedy of the article is that both the author and the women reading the article accept doctor-produced (iatrogenic) penile deformities as normal. They do not question why the penis veers to the side or is bowed, both conditions often being obvious genital abnormalities.

Aside from the perfectly normal variations of the penis (normal bowing and curving), there are only two conditions that result in the erect penis having marked deviations to one side. One condition involves fibrosis (scarring) of the cavernous bodies (Peyronie's disease) which is quite rare. The etiology of this condition is unknown. The second condition causing penile bowing or deviation of the penis off the midline is iatrogenic, (i.e. physician-induced) resulting when too much of the skin sheath is removed during circumcision.

Victims' Voices . . .

"There is no standard on how much to cut off, and even if there was, one cannot judge very well on a baby. When too much is cut off, erections are painful. Too much was cut off of myself, when I was mutilated as a baby."

C.B., Oklahoma

"My situation is as follows. During circumcision, too much skin was removed and the mistake was "corrected" by grafting skin to my penis shaft. The graft was to replace missing skin on the shaft, not to allow for additional skin around the glans. The lessening of sensitivity, while no doubt present at the glans, is most noticeable at the graft site which covers approximately two-thirds of my penis when flaccid and approximately one-third when erect. It also appears that the graft has not allowed for full penis growth as the shaft below the graft is thicker than the graft area itself. I've never been made aware of skin grafting being used to correct misperformed circumcisions."

M.H., Boston

"As is Jewish tradition, I was circumcised at eight days by a man called a "mohel." Apparently, he removed the foreskin further down the penis than was healthy and the error had to be corrected in the form of a skin graft when I was five years old."

M.M., New York

"My grandson was circumcised at birth (sorry to say). I'm told it was not done correctly. He is three years old and he has adhesions, or is it scar tissue. My daughter is hesitant to have it corrected at this time. I wonder if it should be left alone."

Mrs. E.I., Colorado

"My husband had a "radical" circumcision done at birth. We recently discovered this problem, and in conferring with the doctor, found out that almost all his shaft skin was removed, not even enough was left to go around the penis. This lack of skin has caused many problems, including very tight skin over an erect penis."

M.W., San Jose

6. Cleanliness and Hygiene Reasons Mandate That We Do Not Circumcise

- *One is not meant to see the urethral meatus or the glans in infancy.*

- *Smegma is meant to collect under the prepuce.*

- *The circumcised newborn's first perception of genital sensation is severe pain.*

- *Feces and abrasive diapers never touch the glans or meatus of the intact penis.*

- *Following circumcision, there is no way to prevent the glans and meatus from contacting the environment.*

- *"We are aware that a retractable-tip pen lasts longer than one with a permanently exposed ball point, since repeated trauma to the exposed tip renders it functionless long before the ink supply runs out."*

    Leonard J. Marino, M.D.

- *"If it really did offer health benefits great enough to outweigh the injury, it would not be necessary to do it without the consent of the subject."*

    Robert Darby

The definition of circumcision given in practically every dictionary, medical or non-medical, is as follows: "Circumcision: the removal of all or part of the prepuce or foreskin." Many dictionaries add the qualifying phrase, "done for hygienic reasons." Physicians, too, usually include this phrase as their most cogent reason and argument for advocating infant circumcision. It is surprising how naive and unquestioning most people are of these "hygienic reasons." Hygiene is defined as "the science of health and its maintenance," or "a system of principles for the preservation of health and prevention of disease." So let us critically examine this neonatal operation of circumcision that promotes health.

Parents, and most of their doctors, do not know that the preputial space at birth is only a potential space, and that the foreskin at birth is almost always snug, unretractable, and still attached to the underlying glans. One cannot see the urethral meatus (opening) and one is not meant to see the urethral meatus or the glans penis.

American doctors and parents cannot wait for several years, or perhaps until puberty, to see the glans. They must see it "now." After all, "filthy smegma" may be collecting under the prepuce. And everyone knows too that "the foreskin and smegma contribute to venereal disease, cancer of the penis, and cancer of the cervix." If, in the future, "the individual wishes to enter the Armed Forces, he must be circumcised." But most important, "the infant's penis must look like Papa's and like every other boy's shorn penis in the locker room." It is obvious to everyone that the circumcised penis is "cleaner, special, neater looking, unique, and more cared for."

Or is it? If we put all this nonsense aside and examine the hygienic reasons more critically, we discover that hygienic reasons mandate that we do not circumcise.

The prepuce at birth is almost always tight, non-retractable, and adherent to the underlying glans. The delicate glans and the vulnerable urethral meatus are not exposed. This situation persists well into childhood, at least until the child is "out of diapers." Feces and wet abrasive diapers never touch the glans or meatus. This situation is desirable. This is hygienic. This is as God ordained it to be for the infant's well being. Circumcision artificially, prematurely, and deliberately exposes the meatus and glans almost immediately after birth, to an environment that the meatus and glans were not meant to encounter. Following circumcision, there is no possible way to prevent glans and meatal contact and soiling from feces and abrasive diapers. Glans exposure is not desirable; it is not hygienic, and it is contrary to the way it was meant to be. Who is so foolish as to wantonly cast aside this valued protective safeguard of the glans and urethral meatus?

Most Americans understand the value of money, so perhaps a monetary analogy would be in order: Who, after purchasing an expensive camera, would discard the lens cover and then proceed to toss that camera, with its exposed, highly-ground, expensive, delicate lens, onto a shelf, or into a glove compartment, or into a backpack? How long would it take to ruin that expensive lens? Is not the sensitive penile glans—the structure that registers the multitudinous, pleasurable sensory sexual "pictures"—worthy of more care than a camera lens?

There are additional hygienic reasons not to circumcise. The genitals are adjacent to the anus. Any open wound in the area is subject to fecal contamination and possible infection. Numerous infections, including fatal ones, have been documented following circumcision. What sensible person makes an unnecessary, elective incision through the intact skin of a fragile, newborn child in an area close to the anus where it is impossible to prevent fecal soiling of the incision? The thought that an intelligent physician would do this is incomprehensible.

To continue: modified sebaceous glands, the smegma producing glands, are located at the coronal sulcus of the glans penis and at the inner aspect of the foreskin where the foreskin contacts the glans. Smegma serves several extremely valuable functions: It helps dissect the potential space between the adherent prepuce and glans in infancy and childhood; it prevents re-adherence of the prepuce to the glans in childhood; and throughout life, it serves to keep the epithelial covering of the glans smooth, soft, and supple, just as the sebum of our sebaceous glands over our entire body surface keep our skin soft and supple. Our skin becomes rough and dry without sebum. The penile glans becomes rough and dry without sebum. The penile glans becomes rough, dry, brownish, and leathery without smegma (and the protection of the prepuce). One readily perceives this lack of smegma (read: sebum, lanolin, moisturizing cream) if one observes the glans of any older circumcised male. By the time circumcised men reach their thirties, the glans penis has a dry, brownish, leathery appearance. Circumcision destroys a large segment of these lubricating glands, as well as the vehicle for the lubricant's distribution—the mobile prepuce. This destruction of the normal vehicle for constant lubrication of the glans is not desirable nor hygienic.

Certainly accumulated smegma in adults suggests poor hygiene. It is found in children and possibly old men who do not practice proper washing. One does not find noticeable smegma in any civilized man with any intelligence. Gross smegma is readily removed by simple washing with mild soap and water. If one rubs a finger over one's cheek or nose, one appreciates the normal lubricant quality of sebum. So it is with smegma in the sensible male or female. One does not see the smegma, but the glands that produce it are present, and serve to lubricate the glans penis or clitoris, just as sebum lubricates the skin.

The vertebrate animal kingdom would be depleted without smegma. Smegma affects the dissection of their prepuce from their glans and eventually allows glans exposure, and normal sexual function.

6. *(continued)* Cleanliness and Hygiene Reasons Mandate that We Do Not Circumcise

- *What sensible person makes an unnecessary elective incision through the intact skin of a fragile, newborn child in an area close to the anus?*

- *Smegma serves several valuable functions.*

- *Unfortunately most American parents and doctors find penile glans contact with feces more acceptable than the normally occurring, utilitarian glans contact with smegma.*

- *. . . the foreskin at birth is almost always snug, unretractable, and still naturally attached to the underlying glans.*

- *". . . good personal hygiene would offer all the advantages of routine circumcision without the attendant surgical risk."*
  American Academy of Pediatrics

One Woman's Voice . . .

"I did not realize I even had smegma under my prepuce until the age of 45 when I was reading an article on female circumcision and examined myself. No one told me about it, and even as a nurse, I was unaware. In my research of women, I found I am not alone! One hundred percent of the several hundred women I've talked to have never retracted their foreskin to wash—and they have not had problems."

M.M., California

7. No Extra Care Is Needed for an Intact Infant or Young Boy

- *Parents and physicians must get over their compulsion to "do something" to the end of the penis.*

- *Smegma is not "dirty."*

- *Most U.S. doctors are abysmally ignorant about the care of the infant's foreskin.*

- *Forced foreskin manipulation will guarantee problems which will then culminate in the need to circumcise.*

- *The prepuce is a normal structure with a definite function. Like a shoe, a glove, or a hat, it protects the underlying strucutre—in this case, the glans—from the environment.*

- *One washes the child's foreskin as one washes any other part of the body.*

Relevant to a discussion of this topic in the United States, several truisms must be reiterated to the point of tedium: the male infant almost always is born with an attached foreskin which does not permit visualization of the glans nor even the urethral meatus; the foreskin is not meant to be forcibly retracted; smegma is not a "dirty" substance, but a very useful substance that plays a paramount role in slowly and progressively dissecting the prepuce from the underlying glans; the foreskin becomes fully retractable by degrees, over a period of years. It is usually complete by the end of puberty. Neither the parent nor the doctor should retract the foreskin, knead it, stretch or massage it, nor put any probes under it.

In the United States, where most doctors are circumcised and know abysmally little about the foreskin, *it is the responsibility and obligation of parents who wish to retain their son's foreskin to instruct their obstetricians, pediatricians, or family doctors to carefully look at the infant's penis and then, having ascertained its normalcy, to keep his or her grubby hands off the child's foreskin.*

Again, it is not to be pinched, massaged, retracted, probed, kneaded, nor stretched. While most Americans need "instant everything," the normal child, with a normal penis, does not need instant glans exposure. Forced foreskin manipulation will guarantee problems that will culminate in a need to circumcise.

The normal contour of the infant's penis can be accurately ascertained by visual inspection and gentle, non-retractable palpation. One can see the outline of the glans beneath the foreskin. When the infant urinates, there normally is an initial, very brief dilatation of the preputial skin, followed almost instantaneously by the urinary stream. During the remainder of urination, the prepuce remains collapsed. Persistent preputial distention would indicate urinary obstruction at the orifice of the prepuce. This abnormality is uncommon, and can be treated more effectively without circumcising.

Hygienic care of the normal intact penis is perfectly simple. One washes it as one would any other part of the body. Do not retract the foreskin. The inner aspect of the foreskin and the glans are attached, and do not need cleansing. If the foreskin becomes reddened, be a little more solicitous about changing diapers more frequently, or leaving the anal-genital area exposed to the air. One might check the infant's diet (e.g. fruit juice), the nursing mother's diet, the detergent (e.g. bubble bath), or the material in the diaper (e.g. wood vs. cotton fiber). An irritated foreskin is usually caused by ammonia-laden diapers. It is much to be preferred that the foreskin becomes reddened rather than the sensitive glans. After all, this is one of the functions of the foreskin—to take abuse from the external environment rather than subject the glans to abuse.

I had an especially enlightening experience during the several years that I examined the children in my old parochial school. The time was after World War II, when the Russian occupation of Hungary prompted many of the Hungarians to migrate to the United States. In examining the Hungarian children, I found, on occasion, some minor penile problems. The Hungarians do not circumcise their children. In an occasional child in whom I found a phimosis, for example, I would tell the school nurse to inform the child's parents of the situation. Invariably the nurse's note was ignored by the parents. The parents had lived through the Hitler era when an intact foreskin often decided the difference between life and death. The Hungarians are bright, perceptive, earthy people who understand the sexual value of a foreskin. No stupid American physician would induce them into any ridiculous penile operation. The parents knew that with a little more time, the foreskin would become retractable on its own.

In my youth, I swam naked in the streams, the pools of the Y.M.C.A., the Jewish Community Center, and my college pool. Most non-Jews were not circumcised and one could usually distinguish the Jew from the non-Jew merely by looking at the penis. When, on occasion, I swam at the Jewish Community Center, I felt a bit out of place with my prepuce. But then it seemed that those with the permanently exposed glans also felt uncomfortable. I was but an insignificant child at the time and there was never any actual discussion of this matter. I knew then, however, that the glans was appropriately and advantageously exposed upon only three occasions: when urinating, when washing, and when engaging in sex. The constantly exposed glans simply seemed inappropriate.

In the summer, one of our swimming holes was upstream from a public park. Only boys swam there. I often took my dog with me. We never wore suits. On occasion the police would chase us, but we would merely swim over to the opposite bank and hide, and then resume our swimming after the police realized the futility of their mission and left. In the evenings, when the sun went down, we invariably kindled a fire to warm ourselves. In August we would steal corn from the neighboring fields and roast it. After our swim and our corn roast, we had a standard way of extinguishing the fire: We would stand upwind from the fire and urinate upon it. It was kind of neat to hear the fire hiss and sputter as it went out. To get accuracy, maximum force, and distance, one would retract the foreskin and expose the glans and urethral meatus. There was no great mystery about this technique; this was S.O.P.

This putting out of fires by urinating upon them carried over into the entire year. In the fall and winter, we built fires to keep warm, to have fun, and to roast potatoes and apples. In the warmer months we would roast hot dogs and marshmallows. But we didn't need any utilitarian reason to build a fire. We just liked to build fires. And always, if we were not going to use the same location again for our fire, we urinated upon it to put it out.

Another non-sexual thing that we did with our penises when swimming that guaranteed a readily retractable foreskin, was an occasional contest. We would stand in the water, pinch our foreskins closed, and then urinate. The object of the contest was to see who could balloon his foreskin up to the largest size.

We also wrote our names in the snow with our hot urine, and we did have contests to see who could urinate the farthest and the highest.

As I grew older, I was amused at the naivete of the pro-circumcisionists who were so worried about phimosis and difficulty with foreskin retraction of their intact brethren. Their blatant ignorance of the rudimentary principles of penile urinary hydraulics, and the games that little boys play with their penises, were appalling. Possibly in their youth, they should have climbed a few trees, gone swimming in the nude, slept under the stars, and kindled and extinguished a few fires.

Any child with a foreskin knows that if one attempts to urinate without retracting the foreskin and exposing the meatus, the issuing urinary stream will be erratic and unpredictable. One might urinate upon one's clothing, one's shoes, or upon the floor beside the toilet. One does not have to do this very often before one has the common sense to retract the foreskin. Boys and men have known for millions of years that to get predictable accuracy with the urinary stream, one must retract the foreskin. I do not wish the pro-circumcisionists to lose any sleep worrying about this most important issue. Boys and men who have retained their foreskins are retracting them for the above reason and for other cogent reasons.

(Please read "A Father's Voice" on the next page.)

---

7. *(continued)*
No Extra Care Is Needed for an Intact Infant or Young Boy

- *The glans is appropriately and advantageously exposed upon only three occasions: when urinating, when washing, and when engaging in sex.*

- *To get predictable accuracy with the urinary system, one retracts the foreskin.*

- *The likelihood of the foreskin remaining tight and non-retractable is rather remote when one considers how frequently the foreskin is pulled back over a period of time. Assume that the male urinates five times a day, washes himself and his penis several times a week, and masturbates regularly over the course of 10 years, the number of times the boy pulls back his foreskin totals well over 100,000, and this may not even include the times when one is putting out fires!*

7. (continued)
No Extra Care Is Needed for an Intact Infant or Young Boy

- *"Nature is a possessive mistress, and whatever mistakes she makes about the structure of the less essential organs such as the brain and stomach in which she is not much interested, you can be sure that she knows best about the genital organs . . ."*

  Sir James Spence
  Lancet, 1964

- *"The compulsion Americans have for the uncovered glans has provoked a self-fulfilling prophecy: "Those children who are not circumcised have their foreskins forcibly retracted, producing tears, leading to phimosis, requiring circumcision."*

  Genital Abnormalities in the Male

A Father's Voice . . .

"Parents are right to leave the foreskin alone even if it does not separate from the glans for an extremely long time. My parents not only resisted medical advice for circumcision, but also let my foreskin loosen at its own slow rate. I was about 12 before my urethral meatus was visible and 16 before I saw the corona of my glans. Even with this slow loosening of the foreskin, I never experienced irritation or inflammation, contrary to the common medical view of the time that forced retraction of the foreskin was critical to prevent disease. Before becoming sexually active, I spent a few minutes per day over a period of months gradually stretching the foreskin by hand until it would easily retract. This approach was simple, painless, and effective, as well as contrary to the interventionist view that surgery is necessary if the foreskin fails to loosen completely by the time of sexual maturity. There is a wide normal range, and my own experience convinces me that there is no reason to be too quick with the knife.

By contrast, an old-time pediatrician unfamiliar with the need for the child's foreskin to be left alone forcibly retracted our son's foreskin when he was two. Not only was this very painful, causing our son to run in terror to his mother, but led to a temporary build-up of pus. At this point, the pediatrician stated darkly that circumcision would be necessary if the pus continued. We subsequently made sure that our son's foreskin was retracted just for washing, and only as much as he found comfortable. The result was no more pus, no more discomfort, and a penis that is still intact."

H.M., Illinois

8. Your Son Will Learn How Simple It Is to Keep Himself Clean

Physicians and parents commonly mention cleanliness as a reason for circumcising. The circumcised penis is reputed to be cleaner and more readily washable. To use cleanliness as a reason for routine circumcision is both asinine and insulting. The intact penis eventually has a freely retractable prepuce, and anyone with minimal intelligence can wash the entire penis as rapidly, as facilely, and as thoroughly, as one can wash a circumcised penis. The task is no more arduous than washing the middle finger of the left hand. In our literate, affluent society we now possess the knowledge and the facilities to bathe ourselves. It seems a bit radical to substitute a knife and surgery for a little diligent cleaning with soap and water. And to resort to an operation because the average individual—*males only*—may not have intelligence to wash the genitals is a bit ego deflating.

I feel that it's an insult to presume that a child who would grow up to trim his fingernails, blow his nose, brush his teeth, and clean his anus would be too stupid to learn how to retract the foreskin and to wash the glans penis—a procedure no more difficult nor demanding in time than washing a finger. This entire categorizing of males as lacking in common sense relative to penile hygiene is preposterous and insulting. If one can believe the chauvinistic propaganda foisted upon us by the news media, there have even been males who have learned to tie their shoelaces and fly to the moon.

If cleanliness of the genitals were a valid reason for circumcising, it seems incongruous that one should limit the operation to the male genitalia. For in the matter of ease in keeping the genitals clean, the male clearly has the advantage. The male genitals are convex, protruding away from the body, are readily visible, and are relatively far removed from the anus. Except for perspiration and an occasional few drops of urine at the meatus, the genitals are not moist. Urine, of itself, is sterile, albeit slightly malodorous. Of necessity, in urinating, the penis must be held in the hand several times each day. One usually looks at this penis, if only to direct the urinary stream. The male accepts his genitalia as a valuable possession, and normally inspects and handles his penis frequently with little or no feeling of shame or guilt. Certainly a structure that can be readily seen, and is frequently of necessity touched, is more apt to be kept clean than a more inaccessible organ.

In contrast, the female genitalia are more difficult to visualize and cleanse. Madison Avenue warns us of the multiple, malodorous miasms emanating from the female genital tract, and myriads of ridiculous feminine deodorant sprays and douches have been marketed. Actually the anus-vagina-urethra are in close anatomic proximity, and vaginal, urethral, and bladder infections are common. Many women are reluctant to look at, or to touch their genitals. Some have the habit of cleansing their anal areas by wiping forward after a bowel movement, thus soiling their vulvas. Warm, tight, synthetic clothing, menstrual pads, tampons, and vaginal moisture all contribute to difficulties in maintaining perineal cleanliness. The clitoral area is frequently improperly washed, and approximately 20% to 30% of adult females have only partially retractable or actually adherent clitoral prepuces, many with retained smegma.

In truth, the normal vaginal canal has no unpleasant odor, and one needs only resort to sensible washing of the perineal area to maintain perineal cleanliness. Sprays and deodorant douches are superfluous. I know of no one in the United States advocating cutting off any segment of the female genitalia to insure genital cleanliness. It is refreshing to know that surgical procedures are not contemplated for other bodily structures that occasionally have been known

- *It seems a bit radical to substitute a knife and an operation for a little diligent cleaning with soap and water.*

- *In the matter of ease in keeping the genitals clean, the male clearly has the advantage.*

- *The male accepts his genitals as a valuable possession.*

- *The normal vaginal canal has no unpleasant odor.*

- *I know of no one in the United States advocating cutting off any segment of the female genitalia to insure genital cleanliness.*

- *I feel that it's an insult to presume that a child who would grow up to trim his fingernails, blow his nose, brush his teeth, and clean his anus would be too stupid to learn how to retract the foreskin and to wash the glans penis—a procedure no more difficult nor demanding in time than washing a finger.*

9. The Foreskin Is Normal and Natural

- *Every male embryo is genetically programmed to grow a foreskin, and no matter how assiduously we amputate that structure once outside the womb, boys will still be born adorned with foreskins.*

- *The human body is fine the way it is. To try to redesign it, in the absence of illness, is arrogance of the worst sort.*

- *A physician's entire training is geared to distinguishing what is normal and what is abnormal. Disease is a deviation from the normal which one hopes to correct. The normal needs no correction.*

- *"I went to a nude beach in Europe and felt like a freak."*

The subject matter of this book demands that we address the issue of what constitutes the normal. The dictionary says:

1. *Normal*; conforming with or constituting an accepted standard, model, or pattern, especially corresponding to the median or average of a large group in type, appearance, achievements, function, development, etc.; natural; usual; standard; regular.

2. *Biology*; occurring naturally.

Practically every male is born with a foreskin. The male with an anomalous absent foreskin at birth is rare indeed. The foreskin then is clearly normal, and the penis without a foreskin is clearly abnormal. Anatomy texts must include the prepuce in their depiction of what is the normal. Classic paintings and sculpture include it. The seed of doubt about whether the prepuce is a valid normal structure appears to be a uniquely United States phenomenon.

Let us assume then that everyone agrees that the foreskin is a normal part of the male genitalia. Possibly many would argue that its presence is a mistake of nature, but the message apparently has not as yet impacted upon the male's genetic programming.

Whether the foreskin has a significant function is more of a moot question. Most American men and women have had little or no opportunity to evaluate the foreskin and its function. They reject the structure, sight and function unseen.

A physician's entire training is geared to distinguishing what is normal and what is abnormal. Disease is a deviation from the normal which one hopes to correct. The normal needs no correction. At times, the differential judgment is not always so simple, but every time the physician sees a patient, he must make that judgment.

The mission of this book, *Say No to Circumcision*, is to convince the U.S. public that the foreskin is a normal anatomic structure with an important physiologic/sexual function. Removing the foreskin significantly detracts from the sexual experience. The foreskin is responsible for maintaining the sensitivity and function of the penis.

10. What Looks "Funny" to Some Is Natural and Normal

The natural, flaccid penis only looks funny to those who are not accustomed to it. The derisive epithet, "anteater," has even been coined by the unknowledgeable to describe the wrinkled state of the unaroused normal penis. The individual who has never seen a normal erect adult penis must take it on faith that there are no "anteaters" amongst sexually aroused males with normal penises.

The mobility of the penile skin sheath is such that in erection the skin excursion is almost the entire length of the penile shaft, from close to the body to a point beyond the glans. This feature of great skin sheath mobility is exceedingly valuable in facilitating sexual activities, including masturbation, foreplay, and intercourse. In the flaccid state, the natural penis is wrinkled and the skin sheath appears excessive. The glans is hidden, and is in effect, an internal organ. When the penis is fully erect, the wrinkles completely disappear, the preputial skin, in most men, not being sufficient to completely cover the protruding turgid glans.

If one were to be critical of the male's foreskin in its wrinkled state, possibly one should find the wrinkled vulva unappealing. But the male is perpetually and insatiably fascinated by the female's genitalia, despite its wrinkles. And happily, sexual intercourse remains a favorite indoor sport.

Considering the potential physical and psychological harm of neonatal circumcision, as well as the infant's right to own his own body, we must take responsibility for educating ourselves and overcoming our cultural bias with regard to the appearance of the intact penis.

- *The individual who has never seen a normal erect adult penis must take it on faith that there are no "anteaters" amongst sexually aroused males with normal penises.*

- *A prime feature of the normal penis is its exceedingly loose, mobile skin sheath, a quality facilitating sexual activities.*

- *In the flaccid state, the glans penis is an internal organ.*

- *Anatomy books must include the prepuce in their depiction of what is the normal male penis. Similarly classic paintings and sculpture present the naked male with a foreskin.*

Victims' Voices . . .

"I have been in the Unites States nearly five years, since leaving my native Sweden. When I first started dating here, I was surprised, confused, shocked and disappointed because almost all of the men here are circumcised. I have always regarded circumcision as barbaric and ugly. There are many American ways that I still do not understand, and perhaps I am still experiencing a culture shock, but a whole penis can't be that bad, can it?"

Swedish-American woman

"I was circumcised in infancy, and from what I gathered, it only took a few minutes and it was considered a minor procedure. I am now 43 years old and I still suffer every day and night of my life, both physically and psychologically, because of that so-called minor procedure. I will always be my parents' son, but this body that I have belongs only to me and no one else. No one had my permission to circumcise me, and since there was absolutely no medical reason for doing it, it obviously was a clear violation of my basic human rights, and a clear violation of all medical ethics.

If anyone believes in circumcision, then let them be circumcised. But no one should have the right to force circumcision on anyone else. Shouldn't I have the right not to be circumcised if I don't want to be circumcised? Shouldn't I?

Since infant circumcision is a clear violation of human rights and also violates all medical ethics, shouldn't it therefore be outlawed? If we were truly a civilized country, it would be. Remember circumcision lasts a life time, and once done, it's done for life."

G.D., Arizona

10. *(continued)*
What Looks "Funny" to Some Is Natural and Normal

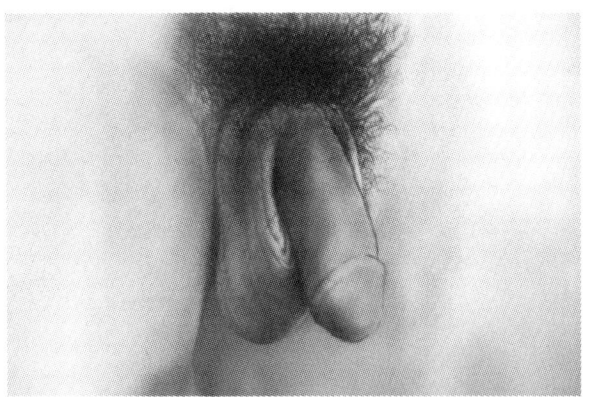
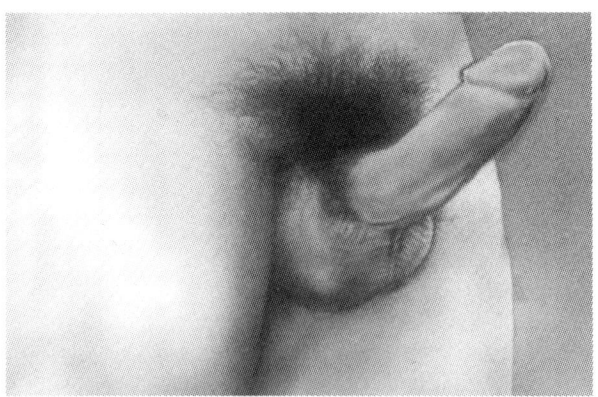

A typical circumcised penis, shown flaccid (left) and erect (right). Note that this is no slack skin on the flaccid penis shaft and the shaft skin is stretched tight in erect state.

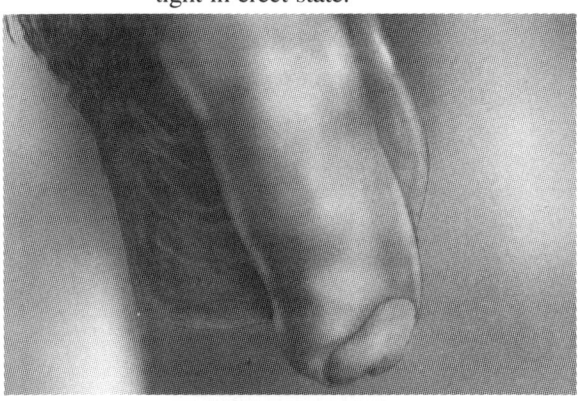
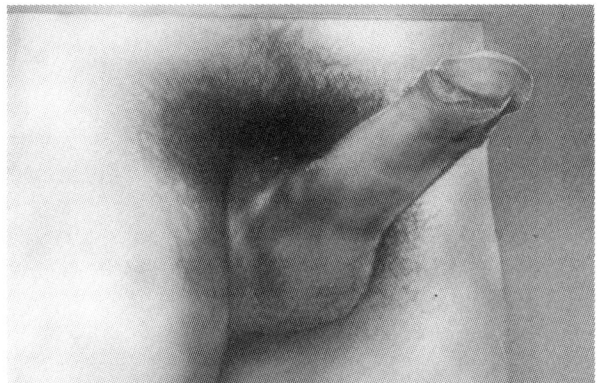
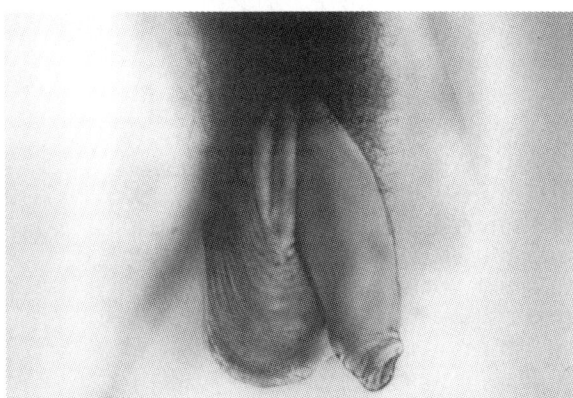
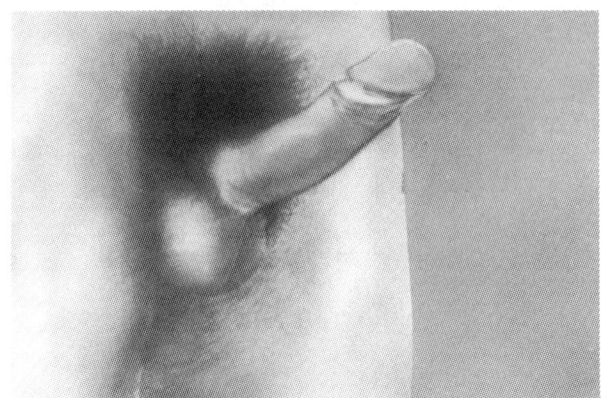

Two typical natural penises, shown flaccid (left) and erect (right). Note the variation of foreskin length in the flaccid state and the relaxed shaft skin in the erect state.

Figure 7.

11. When Unaroused, the Glans of the Penis Is an Internal Organ, Like the Clitoris

The normal glans is smooth, slightly moist, glistening, purple-red, with a mucous membrane surface. It is studded, especially about the corona (the rounded proximal, prominent edge), with multiple, minute, slightly raised, deeper purple-red hemispherical sensory end organs called neuro-vascular corpuscles. Additionally, the mucous membrane glans covering contains numerous free sensory nerve endings. The prominent, raised proximal rim of the glans, the corona, is the most pleasurably sensitive part of the male genitalia. This seems logical since the corona usually has the greatest diameter of the penis, it contains a very great number of neurovascular corpuscles, and the prominent edge is repetitively caught and stimulated by the advancing and retreating foreskin, and/or by the vaginal sphincteric compression mechanism.

The skin is the protective and sensory sheath enclosing the body. The existence of the individual largely depends upon the integrity of this limiting envelope, and through it, exchanges between the environment and the individual take place. At the body orifices, the skin gives way to mucous membrane. Skin possesses accessory structures such as nails, sweat and sebaceous glands, and hair follicles.

Both of these covering structures, skin and mucous membrane, are composed of palisades of cells, with nuclei in the deeper layers, and then becoming flatter without nuclei at the surface. The skin also possesses a coating layer of keratin. The greater the exposure of the skin to abrasion, pressure, and use, the thicker the layer of keratin. Skin is in constant contact with the environment. It is also subject to great temperature variations. It becomes thick when it is subject to rough treatment. The horny (keratinized) layer is thick on the palms and soles even at the time of birth. Pressure and friction at any site provoke it to thicken.

Most mucous membrane normally possesses no keratin layer, sweat glands, hair follicles, nor sebaceous glands. It is softer, usually constantly moist, and its thermal environment usually approaches or is at body temperature. It contacts only selected types of environment, and these only intermittently (for example, the lining of the mouth and esophagus, liquids and food; the nasal vestibule, air of varying degrees of moisture and particulate matter). Independently of hairs, sebaceous glands are present on the inner surface of the prepuce, on the labia minora, and on the areolae of the breasts.

The unkeratinized mucous membrane of the normal glans penis can select its environmental contacts. The normal glans can be an internal or an external organ. The dry, keratinized circumcised glans has no such choice; it is irreparably locked into a condition of constant exposure to a variety of unusual, non-intended, and in a sense, unnatural environmental agents.

Here are some of the major consequences imposed upon the glans penis if the foreskin is amputated by circumcision:

1. The penile appearance is changed forever. The glans is no longer an internal organ and there is no way of protecting it from environmental objects that it was never meant to contact (for example, urine, feces, dry and wet diapers, and clothing). The epithelium (surface) of the glans eventually becomes dry, dull, leathery, brownish, and keratinized, taking on the character of skin rather than mucous membrane. The inner layer of foreskin that produces smegma is removed, thus depriving the glans of its normal moistness and softness. The mechanism for distributing this smegma over the glans—the prepuce—is absent.
2. The recuperative heat mechanism—the foreskin—which maintains the

- *The unkeratinized mucous membrane of the normal glans penis most often is in a protected environment.*

- *The circumcised glans is irreparably locked into a condition of constant exposure to a variety of unusual, non-intended environmental agents.*

- *The protective function of the foreskin is apparent to anyone who has done any small game hunting with a dog.*

- *Altering form alters function.*

- *Circumcision represents a subtraction. The penis has less pleasurable sensory units.*

- *The corona, and **not** the frenulum, is the most sensitive portion of the **normal penis**.*

11. *(continued)*
When Unaroused, the Glans of the Penis Is an Internal Organ, Like the Clitoris

- *In early intra-uterine fetal development, the genitalia of both the male and female have a female appearance.*

- *The numerous sensory units in the diminutive clitoris, combined with the woman's exceedingly short refractory period following orgasm, places the sexually uninhibited female far above any man in the ability to experience sexual pleasure.*

- *Anatomically and functionally, mucous membrane is not meant to be a substitute for skin. The pro-circumcisionists apparently have chosen to ignore this anatomic/functional truism.*

glans at a fairly uniform body temperature, is no longer present to hasten the resolution of minor glans abrasions incurred occasionally in sexual dalliance. In the penis with a prepuce, if any uncomfortable fissures or abrasions occur on the glans, the discomfort can be instantly relieved by drawing the foreskin forward over the glans. The increased heat from the covering prepuce accelerates the healing of minor glans irritations.

3. Certain penile injuries have a greater potential for seriousness in a penis unprotected by a foreskin. In third degree genital burns, the glans and urethral meatus are vulnerable, and any attempt at surgical correction of the burn deformity never produces a totally acceptable result. In the normal penis, the foreskin would take the thermal insult, and the damaged foreskin could be circumcised. The statistical probability of a severe genital burn damaging the glans is much greater than the probability of the individual eventually having a carcinoma of the penis.

4. Circumcision represents a subtraction. One has "less penis." About a quarter to a third of the entire integumental covering of the penis (i.e. skin and mucous membrane) is removed and discarded. The prepuce in itself is very sensitive, so the circumcised male has fewer pleasurable sensory units in his genitals.

5. During infant circumcision, the foreskin is literally forcibly separated from the glans. Some believe this forced separation traumatizes the glans, and may result in desensitizing scar formation. Some glans even exhibit "pits" because the glans is torn away during circumcision.

6. The exposed urethral meatus is subject to constant abrasive trauma from soiled diapers, and after infancy, to the external abrasion of clothing. The meatus often becomes ulcerated and scarred. It loses its normal slit-like opening, and in up to one-third of circumcised children, it becomes stenotic (narrowed), theoretically or actually causing varying degrees of urinary tract obstruction. An operation may be needed to enlarge the scarred meatus.

7. The corona, the most sensitive portion of the entire penis, is damaged, especially because of it's prominence and dorsal location where it is impossible to protect it from clothing abrasion. Its surface, richly supplied with neurovascular corpuscles and free nerve endings, becomes keratinized and less sensitive. Many circumcised males designate the frenulum and not the corona as the most sensitive area of the penis. This may be accurate since the underside of the flaccid penis lies against the warm, moist scrotum where it is sheltered from clothing abrasion. The corona has no such protection. The modern "cod piece," jockey shorts, are admirably suited to deliver this type of abrasive trauma.

Male and Female Comparisons

In any discussion or contemplation of the male and female genitalia, one must remember that, at about the seventh or eighth week of intra-uterine fetal development, the male and female genitalia are at a visually similar undifferentiated state (Figure 8). The genitals in both the male and female fetus have a female appearance. Then if the gonadal chromosomal programming is XX, the genital development continues to be female. However, if the chromosomal imprinting is XY, tremendous changes occur in the male genitalia as a result of the male gonad's input of testosterone. Testosterone causes the female appearing external genitals now to change into those of a male. The greater vulvar lips fuse and form the scrotum. The testes migrate out of the pelvis, and shortly before birth, migrate into the scrotum (the left testis first, and then the right). The lesser vulvar lips fuse and enlarge to form the penile shaft. And almost miraculously, the genitals which appeared female at the eighth week, are now the genitals of a male. This is a truly remarkable transformation.

11. *(continued)*

When Unaroused, the Glans of the Penis Is an Internal Organ, Like the Clitoris

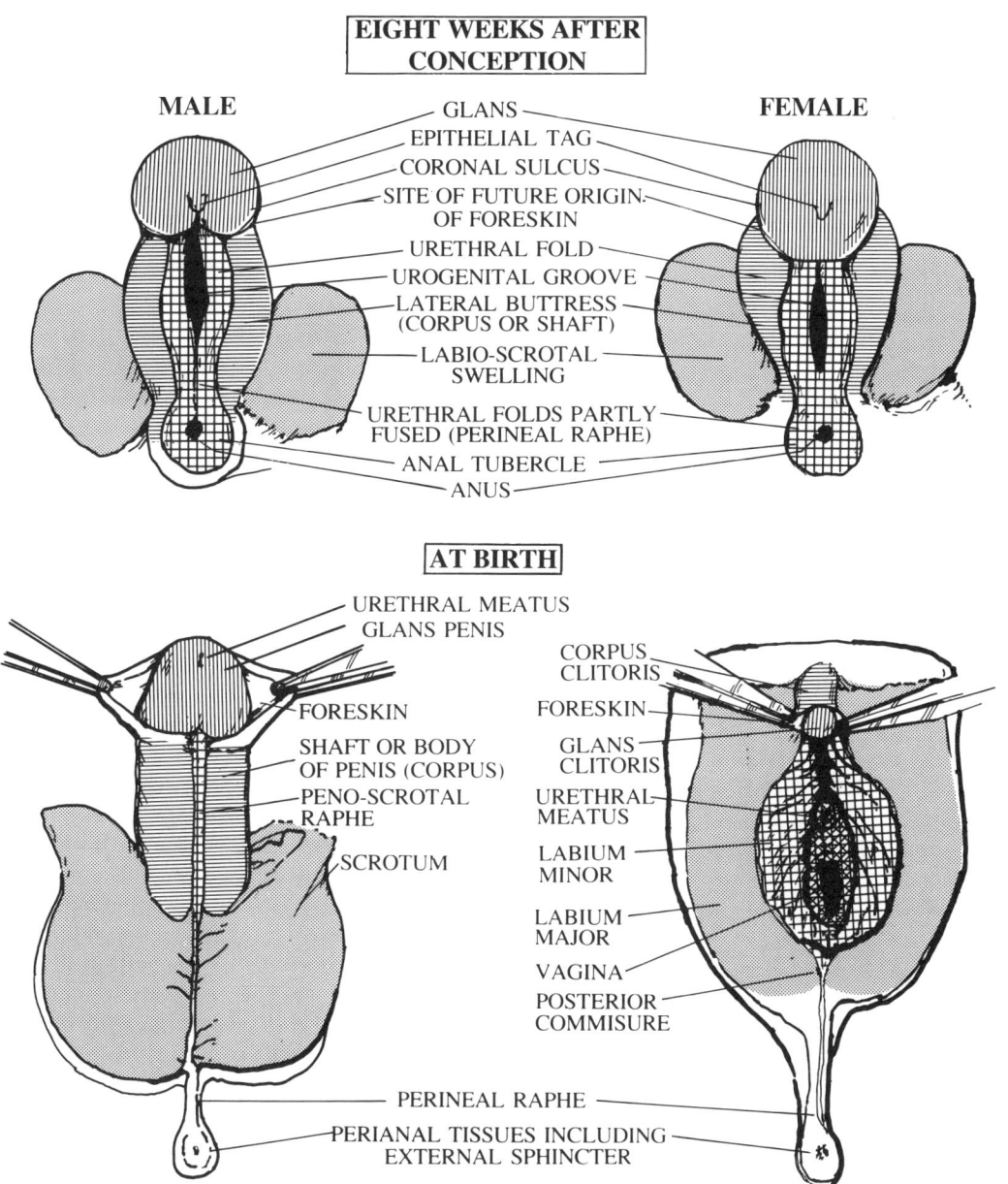

Figure 8.

11. *(continued)*
When Unaroused, the Glans of the Penis Is an Internal Organ, Like the Clitoris

- *So women, who of course are not circumcised, have an inherent pleasure advantage over intact men. And they have an even greater pleasure advantage over circumcised men. This imbalance may not be conducive to a mutually enjoyable sex life.*

At the undifferentiated genital stage, the neural sensory components for genital pleasure "are in place," for both sexes. The number of genital corpuscles and free nerve endings in either the glans clitoris or the glans penis are the same. As the penile glans enlarges, the neural components become more dispersed and diluted. The visually insignificant clitoris, however, remains closely packed with sensory nerve receptors, accounting for its greater sensitivity. This anatomic feature, combined with the woman's exceedingly short refractory period following orgasm, places the sexually uninhibited female far above any man in the ability to experience sexual pleasure. So women, who of course are not circumcised, have an inherent pleasure advantage over intact men. And they have an even greater pleasure advantage over circumcised men. This imbalance may not be conducive to a mutually enjoyable sex life.

Anyone who has gone "barefooted," knows that initially the soles of the feet are very sensitive to the unaccustomed, harsh walking surface. But with time and increased exposure, the sole skin becomes thickened, toughened, and desensitized. A similar toughening and desensitization occurs following circumcision, when the delicate, non-keratinized, moist, sensitive glans is unnaturally and permanently exposed to the harsh environment of diapers and clothing.

12. The Foreskin Enhances Sexual Pleasure!

It has been said that he who does not study and learn from history is bound to repeat the historical mistakes. This apathy applies to any discussion of glans sensitivity in the circumcised versus that in the intact, natural penis. For centuries, circumcision has been viewed as a rejection of the sins of the flesh and as an act of spiritual purification. It has been known throughout history that circumcision makes masturbation and all other sexual activities more difficult and less pleasurable. That's why, in the Western World, it was done by non-Jews.

Dulled Sensations

As recently as the 19th century and the early part of this century, physicians were circumcising in order to dull penile sensation and thus discourage masturbation—a practice that was thought to lead to insanity. It is odd then that people in the United States have so soon forgotten what effect circumcision has upon penile sensation.

As far back as the 13th century, Rabbi Moses Maimonides wrote: "As regards to circumcision, I think that one of its objects is to limit sexual intercourse, and to weaken the organ of generation as far as possible, and thus cause man to be moderate." Some people believe that circumcision is to remove a defect in man's formation, but everyone can easily reply: How can products of nature be deficient so as to require external completion, *especially as the use of the foreskin to that organ is evident*. This commandment has not been enjoined as a complement to a deficient physical creation, but as a means for perfecting man's moral shortcomings.

The bodily injury caused to that organ is exactly that which is desired; it does not interrupt any vital function, nor does it destroy the power of generation. Circumcision simply counteracts excessive lust; for there is no doubt that circumcision weakens the power of sexual excitement, and somewhat lessens the natural enjoyment—the organ necessarily becomes weakened when it is deprived of its covering from the beginning.

Our Sages say distinctly: "It is hard for a woman, with whom an uncircumcised had sexual intercourse, to separate from him. This is, as I believe, the best reason for the commandment concerning circumcision."

And again Rabbi Maimonides advises: "No one . . . should circumcise himself or his son for any other reason but pure faith."

While most people of the Mediterranean were circumcised in ancient times, the Greeks and the Romans were vehemently opposed to the practice. The Greeks preserved the foreskin knowing that it maintained the sensitivity of the glans. The foreskin was also essential to the Greek's sense of modesty, as the bared glans was considered indecent and even obscene—probably because the glans normally is on view only when the penis is erect, which was never in public. Many people today, who have retained their foreskins, have this same aversion to the constantly exposed glans as being ill-mannered and inappropriate, akin to chewing with one's mouth open.

Erection[2]

So the effect of circumcision in dulling penile sensation is nothing new. The ancient Greeks knew, Rabbi Maimonides in the 13th century knew, and physicians around the turn of the century knew.

There is much confusion concerning erection and circumcision. All penises, when erect, are superficially identical in appearance, but upon closer examination, many differences can be noted. There are many myths about the foreskin and erection.

The erect penis with a foreskin is not longer, thicker, or firmer than its circumcised counterpart. However, there is a difference in the distribution and amount of erotogenic tissue.

When erection occurs in the circumcised penis the shaft elongates and

---

- *Physicians were circumcising to dull penile sensation.*

- *The Greeks believed the foreskin maintained the sensitivity of the glans. The bared glans was considered indecent and even obscene.*

- *The glans normally is on view only when the penis is erect, which is never in public.*

- *The effect of circumcision in dulling penile sensation is nothing new.*

- *"Circumcision counteracts excessive lust, for there is no doubt that circumcision weakens the power of sexual excitement, and sometimes lessens the natural enjoyment."*
  Rabbi Moses Maimonides
  1135-1204 A.D.

- *"No one . . . should circumcise himself or his son for any reason but pure faith."*
  Ibid

12. *(continued)*
The Foreskin Enhances Sexual Pleasure!

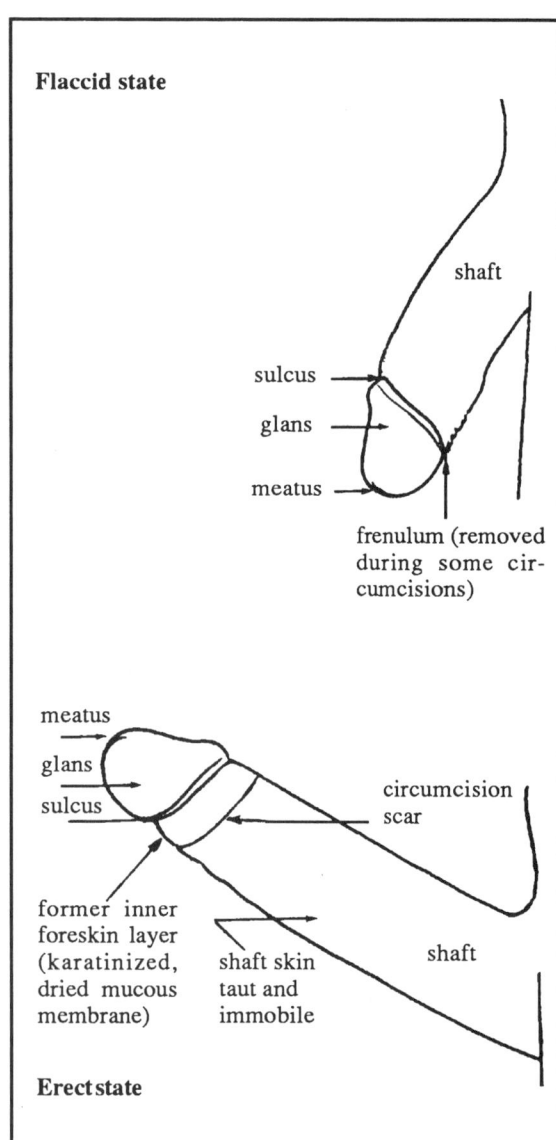

Figure 9. Erection process of circumcised penis

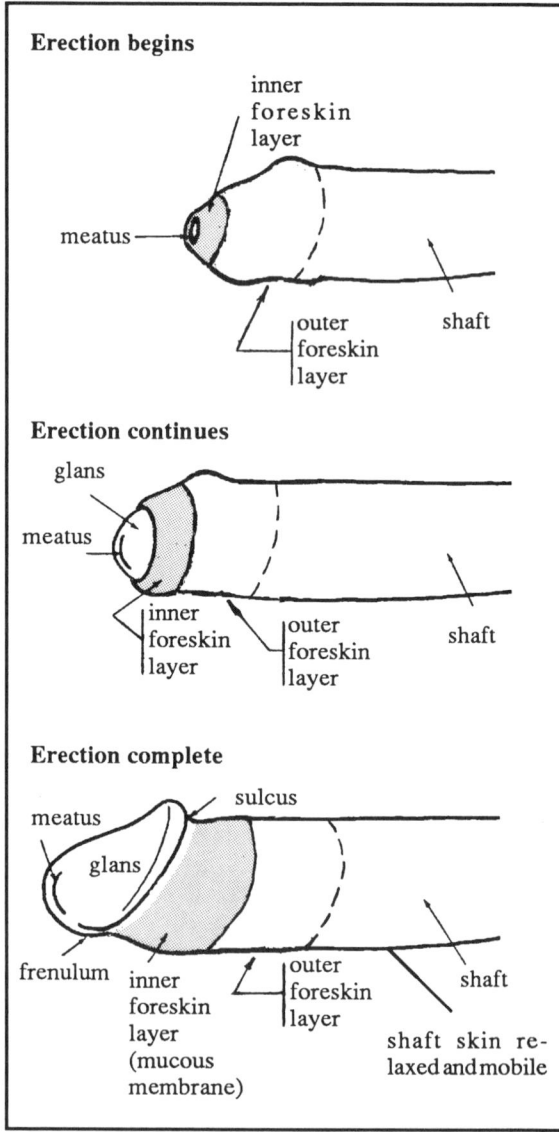

Figure 10. Erection process of natural penis

the shaft skin stretches, being almost taut and fixed at full erection (see Figure 9). However, in the intact, natural penis, as the shaft elongates (see Figure 10), the glans begins to protrude through the opening at the tip of the foreskin, which, since it is soft and pliable, can easily stretch to accommodate the protruding glans. The outer foreskin layer does not shift position; it is the glans that moves outward to extend beyond the foreskin. The outer foreskin, then, no longer covers the glans but remains a continuation of the elongated penile shaft skin. However, since the outer foreskin layer is attached to the inner layer at the tip of the foreskin, the protrusion of the glans causes the inner layer to shift position. The inner layer first slides past the outer layer like a sleeve lining extending beyond the sleeve. The inner layer then folds upon itself, at which point it only covers part of the glans. As the erection becomes larger, the inner layer continues to shift away from the glans, so that by full erection, the inner layer no longer covers the glans at all. At that point, the inner layer becomes a continuation of the penile shaft skin and is now completely exposed (see Figure 10).

In the fully erect intact penis, the shaft is covered by three tissues: (1) the normal shaft skin; (2) the outer foreskin layer (an extension of shaft skin), which formerly covered the glans; and (3) the inner foreskin lining. This means that the erotogenic inner foreskin, which is now exposed and covering part of the shaft, comes into contact with the vagina in intercourse, thus clearly serving to increase pleasure.

Pleasure Dynamics

Last, but not least, are the pleasurable dynamics that take place between the mobile skin sheath and foreskin, and the glans. You see, with an intact erect penis, the foreskin can and does slide over the glans—during masturbation, foreplay and intercourse (see Figure 10). Here is a medical description of the action:

> When the foreskin is retracted, the receding prepuce exerts a mild constricting pressure on the most prominent, sensitive, greatest-diameter-portion of the glans, the corona. Several events occur at this moment: the male is subjectively conscious that his internally placed glans is now externally exposed; the bulbocavernosus muscle, and the other peri-urethral musculature at the base of the penis contract increasing turgidity within the entire penile shaft and especially within the sensitive glans; the neuro-vascular corpuscles of the glans are compressed and then decompressed; the retracting foreskin exerts traction on the frenulum, causing the base of the glans, to which the frenulum is attached, to be pulled in a downward (ventral) direction. This serves to increase the tautness of the epithelium covering the glans, and exerts further compression and then decompression upon the sensory components, intimately integrated within the epithelial covering of the glans. When the foreskin is brought forward again, this entire sequence of events is repeated.

The psychic and physiologic response of the male to this cyclic unit of penile stimulation is exceedingly intense and pleasurable. If one's partner is participating in this maneuver, the pleasure is immeasurably increased. The dynamic, cyclical penile stimulation during intercourse is illustrated in Figure 11.

Circumcision destroys the natural, slick, facile method of penile stimulation. Ironically, many circumcised men do not know what they're missing. In fact, some who have seen this action (in erotic movies, for example) or read about it can't appreciate it. How can intermittent covering of the glans be enjoyable, they ask? Possibly this puzzlement results from the diminished sensitivity of the circumcised penis. But circumcised men, who have restored their foreskin, are thrilled by this "new" form of stimulation.

Let's look at another analogy. The circumcised penis is like a bicycle with the chain removed. How can a man who has never ridden a fully functional bicycle appreciate how much better it is than one that only coasts and rolls. The circumcised penis has no moving parts, approximating a skin covered dowel.

The standard way of masturbating with a normal penis is to move the very

---

12. *(continued)*
The Foreskin Enhances Sexual Pleasure!

- *The circumcised penis has no moving parts, approximating a skin-covered dowel.*

- *But circumcised men, who have restored their foreskin, are thrilled by this "new" form of stimulation.*

- *Two recent books by women document, among other things, the loss of sexual pleasure for women, as a result of a circumcised penis:* Sex As Nature Intended It, *by Kristen O'Hara with Jeffrey O'Hara, and* You Call this Love? *by Lisa Bisque. To learn more, see page 40-8.*

12. *(continued)*
The Foreskin Enhances Sexual Pleasure!

mobile skin sheath forward until it covers the glans and then retracting the sheath to a point very near the body at which point the glans is fully exposed. There is no friction, no lubricant is needed, and the exquisitely sensitive glans itself is not touched except by the sleeve of the moving foreskin. Circumcision destroys this slick, easy, and pleasurable method of penile stimulation.

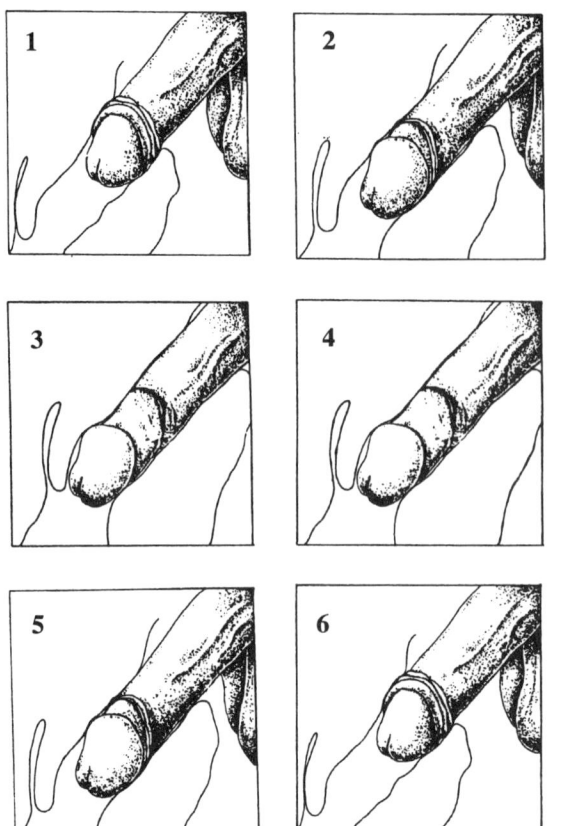

1. The penis begins to move inward.
2. The glans is completely exposed and in contact with the vaginal wall as the penis glides through its unfolding shaft skin.
3. At the end of the in-stroke the sensitive inner foreskin layer below the glans is moving along and in contact with the vaginal wall.
4. The penis begins its out-stroke.
5. The penis moves outward gliding into its mobile skin sheath.
6. At the end of the out-stroke the glans is partially engulfed in the foreskin, or possibly completely engulfed (as would likely be true during foreplay or masturbation).

Figure 11. Uncircumcised penis pleasure dynamics during intercourse

A Victim's Voice . . .

"However, that aside, I am writing to you now with a very clear message—and one that I feel you do not stress enough. The greatest disadvantage of circumcision, in my view, is the awful loss of sensitivity and function when the foreskin is removed. You will recall that I was deprived of my foreskin when I was 26; I had ample experience in the sexual area, and I was quite happy (delirious, in fact) with what pleasure I could experience—beginning with foreplay and continuing—as an intact male. After my circumcision, that pleasure was utterly gone. Let me put it this way: On a scale of 10, the uncircumcised penis experiences pleasure that is at least 11 or 12; the circumcised penis is lucky to get to 3. Really—and I mean this in all seriousness—if American men who were circumcised at birth could know the deprivation of pleasure that they would experience, they would storm the hospitals and not permit their sons to undergo this unnecessary loss. But, how can they know this? You have to be circumcised as an adult, as I was, to realize what a terrible loss of pleasure results from this cruel operation."

R.T., Denver

13. Circumcision Robs the Male of His Birthright— a Fully Functioning Penis

Circumcision is the only operation where the decision to operate is made solely by non-medical personnel—the parents—acting with little or very incomplete knowledge of the anatomy, physiology, medical indications, contra-indications, complications, or consequences of the operation. Unfortunately, the operating physician may only be minimally better informed.

There was a time in my youth when I saw pictures and movies of bodily mutilations such as knocking out of teeth, scarification of the skin, insertion of plugs in the lips, metal rings to elongate the neck, etc., but I felt secure that such procedures, done for reasons of peer pressure, would never be acceptable in the Western World.

Now I know differently. The parental decision to circumcise their infant is based mainly upon emotion and peer pressure. The parents have little comprehension of the disservice that they are doing to their precious infant son. Unhappily, the decision frequently is made with the tacit consent of an ill-informed and/or prejudiced doctor.

What moral or legal right does any parent have to remove a valuable and normal segment of another human being's body? Would it be moral or legal to remove the tip of every male's left little finger, or to knock out a front tooth, because it was fashionable and everyone else was doing it?

A newborn infant is helpless. He cannot defend himself. He entrusts his proper care to your wisdom and kindness. A parent should not violate that trust.

- *What moral or legal right does any parent have to remove a valuable and normal segment of another human being's body?*

- *A newborn infant is helpless. He cannot defend himself. He entrusts his proper care to your wisdom and kindness. A parent should not violate that trust.*

- *"Do you have such a view of nature, and of evolution, that you deny the usefulness of the foreskin, present in all mammals?"*

    George Denniston, M.D.

- *"If anything is sacred, the human body is sacred."*

    Walt Whitman
    The Children of Adam

Victims' Voices . . .

"I have been angry about the subject of infant circumcision for some time. It started when I realized that it was one of the factors in me taking so long to climax with my sexual partner. How could a country that calls itself civilized do such a horrible thing to its little boys? My thought is that parents have no right to consent to unnecessary surgical procedures on their children anyway. It's rape and should be prohibited by law in all 50 states."

S.R., Ohio

"I'm a 42-year-old man who was circumcised in infancy. I still suffer both day and night because of what was done to me. Until the day that I die, I'll probably be in constant discomfort. To me, being circumcised is like wearing a sock with a hole in the end of it and having my big toe protruding from it. I'm constantly trying to pull my sock over my toe. It isn't painful, but it's constantly irritating. (Try it.) As long as anyone (male or female) is forced into circumcision, "civil rights" is just an empty phrase to me."

D.P., Colorado

"In this part of the country they are still doing it in spite of recent insurance changes. All new things start in the West and move eastward, so maybe the anti-circumcision movement will slowly take hold here. Let's hope so! I was routinely circumcised as an infant and have become increasingly envious of those who are natural and dying to know what it would be like "the other way." I definitely believe males should have a choice. As you say, they can always have it done when they are old enough to know, if they so choose. I doubt if many would make such a choice. The more I read about it, the more senseless it becomes. Tonsillectomies have left the fad market years ago. (I had one of those too!)"

W.T., Pennsylvania

14. It Makes Just as Much Sense to Circumcise Baby Girls

- *Is it not a bit demeaning to circumcise the male for "hygienic reasons," for example, because he is thought to be incapable of washing his normal genitals? Suppose the issue were reversed?*

- *"Female circumcision" as practiced in the Third World countries constitutes a devastating mutilation of the vulva.*

- *"I was interviewed by a talk radio host in Copenhagen, Denmark. He asked me if we circumcise infant girls as well. While this may sound peculiar to us, in a country where genital mutilation isn't practiced at all, they don't understand why either of the sexes is mutilated. Maybe pressure from other countries will cause our medical community to reconsider."*

"Mrs. Jones, you've done exceedingly well. And your little baby girl is just fine. I see no reason why both of you cannot go home tomorrow. If it is agreeable with you, we'll circumcise your little girl today. I would like you to sign the operative permit for this procedure. Let me tell you something about female circumcision . . ."

Would you sign the operative permit? Or, would you contact the hospital administrator in order to investigate your physician's competence, sanity and ethics?

Would American parents accept routine neonatal circumcision of the female? Why not? For, in truth, the minute clitoral prepuce (foreskin) is difficult to keep clean, it is often attached to the glans until puberty, and it collects smegma.

A point of female genital anatomy is in order. At the forward part of the vulva, each lesser vulvar lip divides to form two smaller folds, one of which extends above, the other below, the tip of the clitoris. These lip folds join the folds on the opposite side, and form the prepuce (foreskin) on the top of the clitoris, and the frenulum on the underside. Traction on these lesser lips exerts simultaneous pull on both the frenulum and the prepuce, thus indirectly stimulating the glans. All of the following actions—manipulation of the mons veneris (pubic fat pad), traction on the lesser lips, and compression-decompression of the vestibular bulbs lying on either side of the vaginal orifice—*remote* from the glans clitoris—will *indirectly* stimulate the clitoris.

"Female circumcision" not only would expose the glans to toughening abrasion, but would also interfere with mechanisms for clitoral stimulation. Both these same undesirable effects occur following male circumcision. "Female circumcision," however, is almost never done in the United States today, and such an operation performed routinely in the neonatal period, in our present sexual milieu, might well be interpreted as criminal assault or child abuse.

Like male circumcision, the female operation has been widely practiced by Semitic people. Many Islamic peoples, including those in Egypt and the Sudan, still practice the rite. It is believed that at one time the Israelites also circumcised their female children.

The quotation marks bracketing "female circumcision" are placed there for a good reason. Circumcision of the female in Third World and Islamic countries is not just the amputation of the clitoral hood that one might imagine. A number of different types of mutilations have been included under the broader category of "female circumcision." The procedure is veritably a devastating mutilation of the vulva, performed without benefit of aseptic technique or anesthesia.

Infibulation or "Pharonic circumcision" involves the closing of the vagina, accompanied by the excision of the clitoris and labia minora. In the performance of this "circumcision" the forward portion of the vulva, including the clitoris, is transfixed with a metal or wooden pin. The transfixed parts are then drawn forward and cut off with a scissors, or sliced off with a knife. The clitoral remnant is often torn out by the circumciser's fingers. Because of the extreme vascularity of the female genitalia, bleeding is profuse, and sometimes fatal. Infection, including tetanus, is common.

Estimates are that 110 million females in Africa, parts of Asia, and in many Islamic countries have been subjected to this procedure. Cutting out the entire clitoris, as well as removing parts of the small and large vulvar lips, is the most common form of mutilation. It is performed in some 22 African countries alone. Infibulation is the single most popular form of premarital sex deterrence in many Islamic countries.

The operations are frequently conducted in modern hospitals equipped with Western technology and subsidized in part by Western dollars. The U.S. Agency for International Devel-

14. (continued)
It Makes Just as Much Sense to Circumcise Baby Girls

- *Can one with dulled genitals experience the normal full measure of physical and psychic pleasure inherent in the act of making love?*

opment funds facilities in areas where infibulation is practiced. Thus, Washington has become an unwitting accomplice to this act of female genital mutilation.

"The child, completely naked, is made to sit on a low stool. Several women take hold of her and open her legs widely. After separating her outer and inner vulvar lips, the operator slices open the hood of the clitoris and then reaches underneath the length of the clitoris with her finger to detach and pull out the organ entirely. The inner lips are now cut off and the skin from the inside of the large lips is scraped with the knife, so that the lips will eventually seal and narrow the vaginal opening."

The resultant vulvar deformity is tremendous: The clitoris is gone, and large segments of the sensitive lesser lips of the vulva are gone. The bleeding amputated surfaces are either sewn together (infibulated) initially, or eventually they adhere. Only a small vulvar opening remains to permit the passage of menstrual blood and urine. Mechanically the vagina becomes almost impenetrable, and virginity is assured until such time that the woman marries. Then the scarred adherent vulva is reopened on the honeymoon by the solicitous bridegroom, or the circumciser who is called in to do the job.

The procedure serves several purposes: the obtunding (dulling) of genital sensation makes lascivious play and unauthorized intercourse less tempting; a mechanical block to intercourse (the chastity belt concept) is established; and the woman's virginity keeps her a marketable product, retains her status as chattel, and keeps her subjugated to the man. A non-virgin is not marriageable and is a lifelong drain upon the family economy.

Interestingly, infibulation or "Pharonic circumcision," is usually performed by women, upon women, but to serve the convenience and purpose of men. The United Nations Health Organization has had about as little success in abolishing the practice of "circumcision" and infibulation in Third World countries as have the groups of individuals in the United States in ending the practice of routine newborn circumcision of the American male.

Can one with dulled genitals experience the normal physical and psychic pleasure inherent in the act of making love? And is not the partner in that act of love also cheated of the full measure of feedback to which he/she is entitled? This result is one of the profound tragedies of subtractive genital surgery, in either the woman or the man.

So what is the difference between female genital mutilation and male genital mutilation? If what you have just read sounds like torture for the girl, is it not torture for the boy? Part of the genitals are removed without the consent of the individual.

Boy Babies and Girl Babies . . .

"Circumcision advocates most often try to justify the surgery by saying: It decreases the risk of urinary tract infections (UTI's); it decreases the risk of sexually transmitted diseases (STD's); it eliminates the risk of penile cancer; it makes the penis cleaner.

Well, let's give them the benefit of the doubt and assume that these claims are correct (and let's disregard the pain, the complications, and the diminished sexual function caused by circumcision). Then it naturally follows that these assumed benefits can also be bestowed on women through routine infant genital surgery. After all, women's genitals are overlaid with skin folds and are moist—perfect for UTI's and STD's. Cancer of the vulva is much more common than rarely seen cancer of the intact penis. And female personal genital hygiene is surely more complicated than in the male. Is infant genital amputation then the answer for UTI's, STD's, cancer, and cleanliness in the female? Of course not. It is unthinkable!

Then why . . . why do we accept it for males? Physicians and parents must search their own hearts for answers. The next generation of little boy babies is listening . . . and wondering . . . and hoping. How will we respond? What will we do to them? They don't want restraint boards, betadine, surgical drapes, crushing clamps, surgical scissors, excruciating pain . . . They just want to be hugged and cuddled and suckled and loved—just like little girl babies. Just like anybody would want. Can't we do that for boy babies? Can't we *just* do that for them?"

K.H., Illinois

15. Circumcision Is a Disservice to Both the Male and Female—Especially in Later Life

- *Ads for vaginal lubricants are commonplace in current women's magazines.*

- *The circumcised male, because of altered penile function and sensitivity, can never reach his full God-given potential of genital pleasure. The woman, in return, can never be a witness and recipient of her lover's full response.*

The circumcised, erect penis nearly approaches the structure of a dowel. The psychic pleasure of uncovering the glans in sexual play has been denied to the male. The visual and psychic pleasure has likewise been denied to his partner. Traction on the frenulum and its indirect effects on the glans have been spoiled. Indirect stimulation of the glans by the foreskin has been eliminated. The dulled glans can now only be stimulated directly.

During intercourse with an intact penis, the male's mobile sheath is placed within the woman's vaginal sheath. It is impossible to imagine any better mechanical arrangement for non-abrasive stimulation of the male and female genitalia than this slick "sheath within a sheath." Circumcision destroys this.

Several years ago, a toy called the Marvelous Sea Eel was marketed which simulated very nicely how, in a totally non-abrasive fashion, the normal penile skin sheath moves over the underlying erectile bodies. As one securely grasped the covering sheath of this toy, the underlying fluid-filled cylinder readily moved about with no motion (or abrasion) occurring between the encircling hand and the outer cover of the toy.

Circumcised males sometimes need an additional lubricant (e.g., Lubrin suppository, KY Jelly) for non-irritating intercourse. The sheath within a sheath of the normal penis obviates such a need. But the greatest and most tragic result of circumcision is the effect that the altered penile function and dulled sensation have upon the man-woman relationship. The male can never reach his full God-given potential of genital pleasure. The woman, in return, can never be a witness and recipient of her lover's full response. Therefore, she is deprived and cheated out of what she should rightfully share and receive.

One might draw several analogies to illustrate how the altering of penile function and sensation might impact upon the male-female relationship: A gifted musician, despite his/her virtuosity, could not deliver an exemplary performance with a poorly tuned or less than excellent quality instrument; or a gourmet cook married to a man with an impaired sense of taste and smell could hardly expect accolades and full praise for her superior cuisine from a husband who could not fully savor what he eats.

Between menarche (about age 12) and menopause (about age 50), adequate vaginal lubrication at the time of intercourse is usually assured by a combination of factors:

1. Estrogen input—the vaginal mucosa is thick, lush, moist, and resistant to infection and abrasion.
2. "Vascular sweating"—the female counterpart of the male's erection—secondary to sexual arousal.
3. Saliva—that most universally utilized and readily available agent.

Following estrogen withdrawal at menopause, the vaginal mucosa becomes thin, atrophic, drier, and less tolerant of abrasive irritation, especially from a dry, keratinized penis lacking a mobile skin sheath.

Certainly atrophic vaginitis secondary to estrogen withdrawal is the most important factor in the production of dyspareunia (painful intercourse) in older women, but one would be foolish to discount the circumcised male's immobile penile skin sheath as contributing to abrasive vaginal discomfort.

Painful intercourse (dyspareunia) can be remedied somewhat by extraneous lubricants, more gentle love-making, and systemic and/or local estrogen replacement.

In summary, circumcision is a disservice to both the aging male and female. In the older female, dyspareunia (painful intercourse) is more common because of the loss of the mobility of the penile skin sheath, and the subsequent greater abrasion resulting when the dowel-like penis moves in and out of the estrogen-deprived vaginal sleeve.

In the male, drying and thickening of the epithelium (surface) of the glans, secondary to a lifelong exposure to an abrasive environment, decreases sensation and makes obtaining and retaining an erection more difficult.

15. (continued)
Circumcision Is a Disservice to Both the Male and Female—Especially in Later Life

- *"Even an uncircumcised man with bad technique is more satisfying to me than the best circumcised lover. You get that double motion action with an uncircumcised man. It's the best."*

    Woman caller on radio talk show

- *"My newly naked, sensitive glans penis was protected from irritation with cotton and such. Slowly the area lost its sensitivity, and as it did, I realized I had lost something rather vital. Stimuli that had previously aroused ecstasy had relatively little effect."*

    J.T., Los Angeles

Victims' Voices . . .

"I am a 24-year-old male in my second marriage. My first marriage fell apart because of what didn't happen in the bedroom. I was constantly on edge because of sexual frustration. Now, my second marriage is slumping in the bedroom. I have little trouble with erections or ejaculations. My problems are lack of intensity, numbness during and after intercourse, and self-consciousness about the appearance of my circumcised penis."

A.M., Missouri

"Circumcision was virtually unthought of in Wales where I was born in 1922. Since about the time of my entry into the R.A.F. in 1942, I have been reasonably heterosexually active all my life. In 1959, while attending U.C.L.A. as a graduate student, I became friends with a group of Jewish interns and faculty at the University Medical Facility. During this time I contracted a skin disorder around my glans penis. The area became swollen and sore. My foreskin would not retract and sexual activity was difficult. Reporting this to the U.C.L.A. Medical Facility and my friends, I found out that I needed an operation that required the stretching or cutting of the prepuce and subsequent antibiotic treatment. No mention was made of circumcision. An operation was performed, and I recovered clear consciousness to discover that I had been circumcised. Very obviously sincere and intense explanations by my medical friends of the health necessity for the action smothered my irate objections. So it was that I was permanently deprived, and the humorists deflated my complaints.

My newly naked, sensitive glans penis was protected from irritation with cotton and such. Slowly the area lost its sensitivity, and as it did, I realized I had lost something rather vital. Stimuli that had previously aroused ecstasy had relatively little effect. There was a short period of depression, but acceptance of the situation developed, as it had to do. The acute sensitivity never returned, something rather precious to a sensual hedonist had been lost forever. So, it is that I hope you will do what you can to discourage circumcision. My experience and reading indicates that the operation is not only medically unnecessary in the great majority of cases, but also that circumcision destroys a very joyful aspect of the human experience for both males and females."

J.T., Los Angeles

"I became obsessed with the idea that my boyfried should be circumcised. We were very happy together, had much in common, and best of all, we were very compatible in bed. But I refused to get married until he was circumcised—and he gave in.

That little operation completely destroyed our life together. Before he had fabulous staying power, but after the operation he would have an orgasm in five minutes and leave me high and dry.

To make things worse, sex became very painful to me. Twice I had to see a doctor due to minor infections from the chaffing. Our beautiful sexual togetherness became a laborious nightmare of staying creams, lubricants, and frustrations.

He says he will never forgive me, and we no longer speak to each other . . . but I cannot forget what a stupid mistake I made which altered the life of a lovely person."

B.V., Miami

15-2

16. Europeans and Asians Do Not Circumcise Their Sons

- *The United States is the only country in the entire world that routinely circumcises **most** of its newborn males for other than religious reasons.*

- *However, routine newborn circumcision is still an issue in Canada, Australia and New Zealand. The Canadian rate varies greatly from province to province, but experts estimate the overall routine newborn circumcision rate at about 20%. Australia has about a 12% rate, whereas, the rate in New Zealand is significantly lower.*

- *In Canada, there has been a dramatic decrease in circumcisions paid for by Provincial Health systems. In 1975, it was 44%; in 1995, 20 years later, only 4% of circumcisions were paid for by the health system.*

It is significant that the United States is the only country in the world that routinely circumcises **most** of its newborn males for other than religious reasons.

How have the people of Europe reacted towards this neonatal circumcision issue? Surely the Europeans are as knowledgeable as we in matters of public health and preventive medicine. Circumcision is not practiced to any great degree in any country of Europe.

Asians do not practice infant circumcision. And in England, the infant circumcision rate dropped to almost zero when the national health care system did not pay for it. In the 40 years since the practice ceased there, they have not had the dire consequences American medical professionals led us to believe would happen to our sons if we left them intact.

Circumcision "No"

Just **some** of the countries that **do not** practice routine medical infant circumcision:

Western Europe
- Belgium
- Denmark
- England
- France
- Finland
- Germany
- Ireland
- Italy
- Netherlands
- Norway
- Portugal
- Scotland
- Spain
- Sweden
- Switzerland

Eastern Europe
- Albania
- Austria
- Bulgaria
- Czechoslovakia
- Greece
- Hungary
- Poland
- Romania
- Russia
- Yugoslavia

Asia
- China
- Korea
- Philippines
- Japan

Central America
- Costa Rica
- El Salvador
- Guatemala
- Honduras
- Mexico
- Nicaragua
- Panama

South America
- Argentina
- Bolivia
- Brazil
- Chile
- Colombia
- Ecuador
- French Guiana
- Guyana
- Paraguay
- Peru
- Surinam
- Uruguay
- Venezuela

Circumcision "Yes"

All of the countries that practice routine medical infant circumcision on a **majority** of their males:

U.S.A.

17. The "I'm Circumcised and I'm Fine" Syndrome

Many fathers lean towards circumcision for their newborn sons based on the erroneous logic expressed in the statement, "I'm circumcised and I'm fine." From the father's point of view he is fine. His penis is erect when required and it provides significant pleasure. But can the typical circumcised man trust his point of view to lead him to the right conclusion in judging whether he is actually "fine"?

The answer to the above question is "probably not," and here's why. First, the typical circumcised man has no means of accurate comparison—after all, he's been circumcised all his life. All of his sexual experience has been with his circumcised penis. If a person, color blind for life, didn't learn what colorblindness meant, he would think the colorblindness was normal. And, in fact, he would think that it was "fine."

Second, the average American man is woefully lacking in knowledge about the functions of the foreskin, glans sensitivity and the pleasure dynamics (see Chapter 12) of the normal intact penis. This is not surprising, since the medical community and consumer medical books have not made this information available. You might say, "Well, shouldn't men find out these things in the locker room or from their buddies?" It would be nice if they did, but it doesn't work this way because men don't talk with other men about penises, and anyway, the vast majority of adult men are circumcised so they wouldn't know anything anyway. And intact men are often intimidated by the "majority" so they do not share their personal knowledge.

The third and final reason is possibly the most compelling. Circumcised men are by the very state of their penises trapped into a biased position. Everyone wants to think they're "fine," especially when it comes to those attributes that they cannot change. The penis is the typical man's most cherished physical possession. To admit that it is not all that it could be takes a great deal of soul searching and intellectual honesty. And this admission brings on deep feelings of anger and frustration, because the deficiency is not natural (i.e. like a birth defect) but was inflicted at birth by a misguided physician and ill-informed parents. Denial is a common defense mechanism. Maybe it's most common of all among circumcised men.

One perspective that may be enlightening is that of men circumcised as adults. Please read the Victim's Voices below for this insight. These circumcised men do not think their altered penises are "fine"!

■ *"I have the greatest respect for those fathers who, having been circumcised themselves, refuse to have it done to their sons."*

George Denniston, M.D.

Victims' Voices . . .

"After thirty years in the natural state, I allowed myself to be persuaded by a physician to have the foreskin removed—not because of any problems at the time, but because, in the physician's view, there might be problems in the future. That was five years ago, and I am sorry I had it done now from my standpoint and from what my female sex partners have told me. For myself, the sensitivity in the glans has been reduced by at least 50%. There it is unprotected, constantly rubbing against the fabric of whatever I am wearing. In a sense, it had become calloused. Intercourse is now (as we used to say about the older, heavier condoms) like washing your hands with gloves on . . . I seem to have a relatively unresponsive stick where I once had a sexual organ."

S.J., Denver

"Orgasm, which I feel as deep muscular sensations, has not changed but my perception of intercourse is very different. Sharp, strong sensations from the surface of my glans and upper shaft have given way to much duller sensations of pressure and warmth under the skin."

T.B. (circumcised as an adult)

"The sexual differences between a circumcised and uncircumcised penis is . . . [like] wearing a condom or wearing a glove . . . sight without color would be a good analogy . . . only being able to see in black and white, for example, rather than seeing in full color would be like experiencing an orgasm with a foreskin and without. There are feelings you'll just never have without a foreskin."

R.G. (circumcised as an adult)

18. Circumcision Removes A Lot More Than a Little Snip of Skin

- *Circumcision removes a piece of skin almost equivalent to a 3 x 5 inch index card.*

- *Circumcision removes one half or more of the entire skin of the penis—a tragic loss of erogenous tissue.*

Sure infants' penises are small. Their whole being is small. But a 7-pound, 18 inch, baby grows into a 6-foot 2-inch man. And that very little penis grows up too. And so does its foreskin. In fact, the foreskin, as measured on adult males, is surprisingly large. Remember, the foreskin on a flaccid penis goes from the base of the glans penis out past the tip of the glans, and then folds back on itself and returns to the base of the glans. Pathologists have measured the average foreskin to be about 2.5 inches in length—from its base, out to the tip, and back again.

And, of course, it surrounds the glans which is about 1.5 inches in diameter, or about 4.7 inches in circumference. So the entire skin surface area of the average adult foreskin is almost 12 square inches! That's equivalent to a piece of skin almost the size of a 3 x 5 inch index card.

The average erect adult penis is 6 inches in length, with a shaft of about 4.5 inches. So the shaft skin of the circumcised penis when it's all stretched out is about 21 square inches. This means that foreskin amputation of an infant results in the loss of a third or more of the adult's total penile skin covering. How sad and tragic. And let's not forget, the inner portion of the foreskin is sensitive, erogenous mucous membrane.

Circumcision Skin Removal

Note: The area of the box above (15 square inches) is about the same as the surface area of the average adult foreskin.

19. Your Son's Penis Does Not Have to Look Like His Father's

What psychic trauma would be inflicted upon your son if his father had black pubic hair, a pot belly, an appendectomy scar, and his right testicle hung lower than the left. And your son's pubic hair was brown and he had a nice flat abdomen without a surgical scar, and his left testicle hung lower than the right? Would you seriously consider having your son or husband consult a plastic surgeon so that their genitals and lower abdomen would more closely approximate each other in appearance? Is one's psyche so fragile that one must have clones of the genital area of one's parents and/or siblings?

While it is true that most males surreptitiously, visually "check out" the other naked males' equipment in the locker room and soon discover that "all men are not created equal," one seriously doubts that the inequality in the appearance of the end of the penis has produced any rash of mental breakdowns.

I'm of an age when most men had penises unaltered by circumcision surgery. When circumcision became the order of the day, I don't recall males in my age bracket jumping out of windows or rushing to a surgeon to have any genital tailoring.

This entire compulsion to have "my penis look like Daddy's, and to have tunnel vision concentrating on the end of the penis, seems exceedingly bizarre. Could it be that the father who is circumcised is the one whose psyche is disturbed when he contemplates his infant son's normal penis? Knowing that his own penis was altered for the worst, at a time when he had no choice in the matter, would the father, out of a feeling of jealousy and envy, consent or suggest circumcision so that his little son's genital status would not surpass his own?"

Let us be thankful, and rejoice at our little baby's normalcy. He is his own unique person entitled to his own abilities, dreams, aspirations, and appearance.

- *Anatomy books, statues and paintings depict the naked male with a prepuce.*

- *Americans now view the constantly exposed glans as the normal.*

- *"What was so difficult in leaving my son intact was not that my son would feel different in a locker room, but that I would feel different from him. I would then have to accept that I'm an amputee from the wars of a past generation."*

  A Father's Lament

- *Let us be thankful, and rejoice at our little baby's normalcy. He is his own unique person entitled to his own abilities, dreams, aspirations, and appearance.*

Victims' Voices . . .

"Sad to say I also was a victim at birth. Too bad babies cannot fight back, but then that is why they are perfect for something as brutal as circumcision. I have a 7-year-old son who is perfectly normal and happy with a foreskin."

F.M., California

"I would sell my soul to the Devil ten times over if I could get my foreskin back again. I have two sons who sport two magnificent long, loose foreskins, the sight of which, turns me green with envy. I had to defend their foreskins and their right to retain them, almost with violence, such is the circumcision mania among doctors. God made men's penises with foreskins because they are supposed to have one and I want mine back."

M.G., Maine

"I had my son butchered because of peer pressure 15 years ago. How dare doctors perform unnecessary operations just because they felt Billy was going to be too lazy to keep himself clean! I've heard a man loses 25% of his feeling because of this. That's a lot to take away from someone. I told my wife we could take her to a doctor and get 25% of her sexual feeling taken away. Of course she didn't want such a thing. But neither do I. I'll never forgive myself for butchering my son, and I intend to apologize to him one day soon. Thanks for letting me get this off my chest to someone who understands."

D.A., Pennsylvania

"Just because someone was cruel to my husband when he was a baby doesn't mean I have to perpetuate that cruelty on my son."

L.T., Florida

20. Men Circumcised as Infants Are Even Now Restoring Their Foreskins

- *For more information read "The Joy of Uncircumcising" by Jim Bigelow, Ph.D.*

- *Doctors Opposing Circumcision approves of foreskin restoration. We recognize that an important part of the body has been lost, and that it is perfectly reasonable to want to attempt to restore it as much as possible. We also recognize that a support person is important during the process. We recognize that many doctors fail to support men who ask for help during this process. Indeed, they often ridicule them. We assert that this is inferior medical care. However, since the doctors are victims themselves, it is to be expected. We recommend that men who wish to restore not consult a doctor unless they are certain that he or she will be supportive, and knowledgeable. We recommend non-surgical stretching techniques, rather than surgery that may include grafts. At present, there are few doctors in the US capable of performing this type of surgery to the satisfaction of the individual with the loss. The ultimate solution to this problem is to eradicate the tragic practice.*

Undoing the damage done by circumcision has been attempted in one way or another for several millennia. The Jews, for example, who engaged in the Greek Olympic Games, in which the contestants were naked, tried to hide their exposed glans penis in many ways and with varying degrees of success. There are several reasons for restoring the foreskin:

Cosmetics—Many people feel that the penis looks better in its natural state without the deformity of circumcision.

Psychologic—Although the glans penis is seldom on public display, the individual feels better knowing that genitally he is all there.

Sensitivity—Circumcision, as stressed repeatedly in this book, desensitizes the glans penis. A significant amount of sensitivity can be regained by recovering the glans.

Sexual Manipulation—The normal intact penis is a better penis with more options for a variety of manipulations in solitary, or during love making. The circumcised penis is simply inferior.

The issue under consideration here is not the variety of reparative techniques—which are bound to change from time to time—but the cost and aggravation involved in order to restore the appearance and function to a structure that initially was normal and which should not have been operated upon in the first place. This restorative surgery also costs lots of money, and non-surgical techniques are often time consuming. But despite meticulous efforts, the normal foreskin can never be totally duplicated. Happily, men who have restored their foreskin, both surgically and non-surgically, report much increased sexual pleasure and a sense of wholeness.

Victims' Voices . . .

"I've been restoring for almost two months and it's hard to believe. But sex with my wife is getting better. I actually have more feeling. It's great."

35-year-old man

"After the coverage, I noticed that I was getting more, let's say, `delicious' feelings during sex with my wife."

57-year-old man

"I have even gone so far as to use condoms—a tedious, time-consuming task on myself to simulate a foreskin; so strong the desire to know what all of my original parts would feel like."

F.O., Seattle

"Infant circumcision has turned out to be a personal tragedy for me. At 37, my circumcision scar is the largest and only immediately apparent scar anywhere on my body. I'm resentful, upset, angry, and now embarrassed about being circumcised because it is a living symbol of senseless violence, oppression, ignorance, and greed, which I have been forced to carry on my body for 37 years. The more I ponder my own circumcision and that of others, the more my heart and mind rage against it. I'm grieving for myself and others who were, are, and will be violated in this way. Infant circumcision is to me a truly vile practice defying all compassion and reason.

I have experienced continued sexual sensitivity problems. During the AIDS crisis I have worn a condom which has proven to make any climax I have expected impossible. After a few weeks of practicing a method of foreskin restoration, I'm convinced that my main problem was circumcision in combination with friction from clothing because I have lived a very athletic lifestyle for many years. The constant friction probably further desensitized me. I was able to completely cover my once barren glans with skin during about the

Victims' Voices (continued)...

second week and noticed suddenly that a major irritation was gone. Since then, other improvements have occurred. The color and texture of my glans has changed to more nearly match the rest of me, and its crevices and callouses are less apparent each week. The glands in the area have begun to produce normal lubrication, and my nose at times catches a faint whiff of natural male aroma, which rather than being unpleasant, is pleasantly reassuring. Now I cannot leave my glans uncovered because clothes irritate it so much that I am unable to endure it for long and develop inappropriate erections from the friction if I move around too much. I can conclude from my experience so far that the normal covered or intact state is greatly superior to the uncovered or circumcised state for almost any human male. I feel that anyone who says that infant circumcision has no negative lifelong effects or is 'minor surgery' is either ignorant or lying, perhaps both.

What will be the future social implications of infant circumcisions done in the next few years? What will be a boy's reaction when he discovers through contacts with intact boys that a major piece of his anatomy is missing for no apparent reason? I feel that when such a person learns the complete truth it could potentially weaken or destroy family relationships. Even I at age 37 think considerably less of my parents because they could have said 'no' to the doctor. My cousin born at almost the same time I was in the same hospital kept his foreskin, and my parents could just as easily given the doctor the same 'no' for an answer. The resentment, anger, and grief reaction of a male who was circumcised without his consent is normal, and the parent who said 'yes' probably deserves 100% of the wrath because that parent is not an innocent party to the action. Intact foreskins could in many instances add up to intact family relationships when boys grow up."

L.R., Ohio

"At this time, I'm able to pull the skin just past the tip of the glans when I'm not erect. When I am erect, the skin can be pulled forward to cover three-quarters of the glans. Most of the time, I'll wear the skin forward, being held in place with the end of a small rubber. I can't tell you how much more comfortable it is that way rather than with the glans exposed. It feels `natural,' `warm,' and protected. I feel whole again as opposed to feeling naked with the glans exposed. Also, you know its funny, but being able to have my skin in either position, I never realized how sensitive the glans is until I wear the glans covered and its protected from rubbing against clothing, etc."

B.A., New York City

"I am a 28-year-old male and I wish to inquire about the possibility of reconstructing my foreskin. I was circumcised at birth, and finally learned at age 16 what circumcision was. I was appalled that this had been done to me. The one part of my anatomy that nature had intended to be truly intimate had been stripped away in some archaic ritual. I feel that I have been disfigured in both my appearance and the mechanics of sexual intercourse. I realize that nerves cannot be mended, but I feel that it may be possible to regain some of the intimacy I have lost."

K.J., California

"Being circumcised at birth, I feel that I was mutilated, and my natural image was altered without consent. That's why I am writing to you now. I have heard about foreskin restoration, and I would like to learn as much as I can about it. I am very interested in restoring what was taken from me."

R.K., Ohio

"I've suffered for a great many years with problems associated with an exposed glans penis and I have finally decided to seek help."

J.D., Carmel, California

"Please send me information on foreskin reconstruction. I am 31 years old. I have been trying to make my penis look `normal' for 15 years. I am afraid that if I confronted `any old M.D.' with the problem, he'd `lock me up.'"

S.A., California

"Help. I was mutilated as a baby. I am considering restoration and would like to obtain all the information you have on both surgical and non-surgical techniques."

M.B., New York City

20. (continued) Men Circumcised as Infants Are Even Now Restoring Their Foreskins

Publisher's Note...

As a service to circumcised men, Hourglass Book Publishing published *The Joy of Uncircumcising: Restore Your Birthright and Maximize Sexual Pleasure*. Write for information to UNCIRC, P.O. Box 52138, Pacific Grove, CA 93950, or call (831) 375-4326.

21. Males with Foreskins Will Have A Lot of Company in the Locker Room

- *The male with the normal penis need feel no reticence in exposing himself to his circumcised peers. He knows that his normal penis did not have to be surgically altered, and that he has been endowed with enough intelligence to master washing the prepuce.*

- *Conversely, the circumcised male need experience no psychic trauma when perusing his intact peers. After all, his surgically altered penis was a result of thinking that was considered proper at the time.*

- *Peer pressure is no sensible reason for the continuation of the operation. Other bodily mutilations—binding of feet, piercing of noses and lips, binding of skulls, knocking out of teeth, infibulation of the female's genitalia, burning and excision of the clitoris—have all been perpetuated on the basis of peer pressure.*

Not too many years ago, newborn infants were fed with formula-milk substitutes. Breast feeding was not suggested nor encouraged by either society in general, nor specifically by physicians. The practice was considered vulgar and animalistic, and nursing an infant in a public place was in very bad taste. Then someone made a most remarkable discovery: Human babies could be fed and would flourish on human milk. Rather quickly, the trend to nurse from the breast "caught on," and today many women breast feed their infants.

A similar about face surely and inevitably is occurring with respect to circumcision. The American public is discovering that the normal foreskin is an exceedingly valuable appendage that needs no meddlesome desensitizing, defunctionalizing surgery.

Similarly, boys do not need to be circumcised just because some child down the street is circumcised. Fortunately, with the current decline in the U.S. circumcision rates, this excuse is less valid than it ever was. The chances are approaching 50/50 that the boy next door is intact, and the locker rooms of the 1990s will reflect that. The normal intact penis is once again assuming par excellence status in the locker room.

"Isn't everyone circumcised?"[6] Every so often you'll hear a circumcision advocate claim that "everyone is circumcised." This is categorically false, and it may also be an attempt to put pressure on American parents to consent to medically unnecessary surgery on their youngsters.

The truth is most males are intact (non-circumcised). Over four of five males in the world are intact and glad! The United States is the *only* nation left which still circumcises a majority of infants *without* medical or religious reason.

Even in the United States, over one-third of our males (40 million men) are intact, while two-thirds (75 million) lost part of their penises shortly after they were born. Although hospital circumcision was promoted in the early 1900's as a "cure" for everything from alcoholism to masturbation, it did not catch on as a "fad" until now–discredited claims were made around World War II that it would "prevent" venereal disease and cancer. Today we know better.

Since the medical community declared in the 1970s that there are no health, cleanliness, or medical reasons to subject babies to the risk of circumcision, the rate has been declining in the United States, especially among knowing parents and those who prefer natural, non-medicated childbirth and minimal pain and trauma for the baby.

The National Center for Health Statistics reports that 59% of the almost two million American boys born in 1993 were circumcised at birth, a decline from the estimated high of 80% to 90% in the 1970s. The figures vary from community to community, often de-

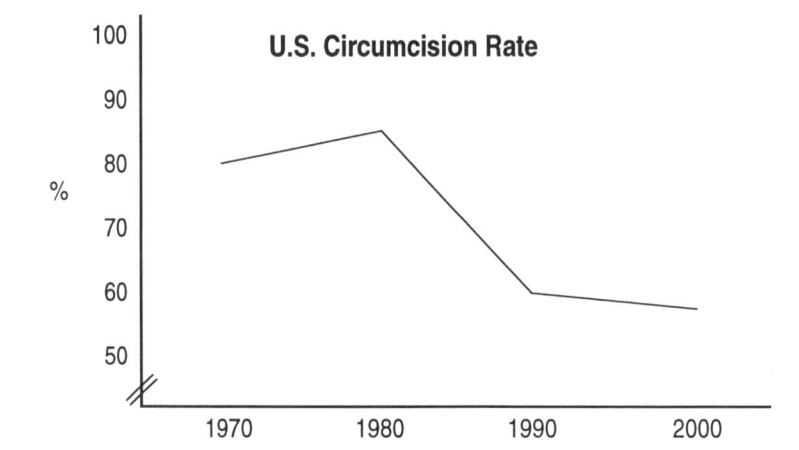

pending on how educated and conscientious the doctors and the hospital staff are in discouraging unnecessary and harmful surgery.

Circumcision rates in 1996, the most recent data available, also vary in each part of the country and are as follows (National Center for Health Statistics):

Northeast	67%
Midwest	81%
South	64%
West	35%

In the western states, where 65% of the boys are now intact, the locker room scene has reversed. Circumcised boys have already begun to ask "Why am I different?" and "Why did you let them cut off part of my penis?"

Whether a man is circumcised or not has nothing to do with his abilities or contributions to society. Most males had no control over whether they were circumcised or left intact. For a number of years, parents were told that circumcision was the medically right thing to do. Now we know better, and *knowledgeable parents leave their boys intact.*

Although one-third of American males and the vast majority of the world's males are intact, some *prejudiced* people in America still suggest that "it is easier for a circumcised boy to grow up and become successful." *This is obvious nonsense,* but some people still pressure parents to circumcise by playing on parental fears. Fortunately, in a pluralistic society like ours, both intact and circumcised boys can grow up together with an equal chance to reach their goals.

Not surprisingly, almost all foreign actors, athletes, and celebrities are intact. A Los Angeles researcher published a list of 20th century celebrities and their circumcision status.[3] *Almost all foreigners on the list are intact* including Prince Albert, Mario Andretti, Mikhail Baryshnikov, Boris Becker, Bjorn Borg, Pierce Brosnam, David Bowie, Michael Caine, Sean Connery, Donovan, Julio Iglesias, Elton John, Ivan Lendl, Peter O'Toole, Sting, all the Beatles, and Prince William (heir to the British throne) and Harry.

The following is a *partial list of intact 20th century American celebrities* excerpted from a list referred to in the previous paragraph.

Alan Alda	Magic Johnson
Paul Anka	James Earl Jones
James Arness	Gene Kelly
Eddie Arnold	Robert Kennedy
Orson Bean	Jack Kerouac
Dan Blocker	Martin L. King
Vida Blue	Perry Kin
Sonny Bono	Jack LaLanne
Marlon Brando	Burt Lancaster
Johnny Carson	Jerry Lee Lewis
Johnny Cash	James MacArthur
Maxwell Caulfield	George Maharis
George Chakiris	Ed Marinaro
Michael Cole	Dean Martin
Chuck Connors	Lee Marvin
William Conrad	Johnny Mathis
Jackie Cooper	Ed McMahon
Francis F. Coppola	Eddie Murphy
Bill Cosby	Bob Newhart
Walter Cronkite	Nick Nolte
Bing Crosby	Hugh O'Brien
Tony Danza	Jack Paar
Anthony Davis	Jack Palance
James Dean	Luke Perry
John Dean III	Jim Plunkett
Jack Dempsey	Elvis Presley
John Denver	Vincent Price
Gerard Depardieu	Charlie Pride
Leonardo DiCaprio	Anthony Quinn
Joe DiMaggio	Ronald Reagan
Buddy Epsen	Robert Redford
Carl Eller	Steve Reeves
Erik Estrada	Burt Reynolds
Don & Phil Everly	Little Richard
Lou Ferrigno	Cliff Robertson
Clark Gable	Mickey Rooney
Joe Garagiola	David Selby
Ben Gazzara	Tom Selleck
Boy George	Frank Sinatra
Frank Gifford	Tom/Dick Smothers
Robert Goulet	Tom Snyder
Peter Graves	Mr. T
Andy Griffith	Robert Taylor
Hugh Hefner	Daniel Travanti
Jimi Hendrix	Al & Bobby Unser
Charlton Heston	Dick Van Dyke
Paul Hogan	Alex Van Halen
William Holden	Eddie Van Halen
Anthony Hopkins	Robert Vaughan
Ron Howard	Jan Michael Vincent
William Hurt	Dennis Weaver
Jeremy Irons	Flip Wilson
Jesse Jackson	Cale Yarborough
David Jannsen	Steve Yeager
Don Johnson	

21. *(continued)* Males with Foreskins Will Have A Lot of Company in the Locker Room

- *The chances are approaching 50-50 that the boy next door is intact, and the locker rooms of the 1990s will reflect that.*

- *The National Center for Health Statistics reports that 59% of the almost two million American boys born in 1990 were circumcised at birth, a decline from the estimated high of 80% to 90% in the 1970s.*

- *Not surprisingly, almost all foreign actors, athletes, and celebrities are intact.*

22. Males Masturbate Whether They Have Foreskins or Not

- *After circumcision, masturbation becomes more difficult and contrived.*

- *But the ingenious male—circumcised or not—will find ways to masturbate!*

- *"The only way to stop masturbation is coma."*

  Leonard Marino, M.D.

Many years ago, an old nun who resided in a nearby boys' orphanage dragged two forlorn little boys into my office. These two young rascals were unlucky enough to be caught "abusing themselves." The nun was intent upon remedial action and she asked me to circumcise the culprits. Foolishly, I complied.

The point of this anecdote is this: This not-so-sexually-naive old nun knew enough about human sexuality to realize that the foreskin facilitates sexual dalliance. But she assumed (wrongly) that the procedure would curtail the boys' sexual activities.

But males masturbate whether they have foreskins or not. Early in infancy the child discovers that fondling the genitals is pleasurable. This activity may well continue throughout one's lifetime. Masturbation is a normal phenomenon and the only harm in its performance is the unnecessary elicitation of guilt and/or shame. In addition to the pleasure it brings, it has the very important utilitarian function of keeping the individual sexually conscious, an attribute vital to the propagation of the human species.

Masturbation is done by either *direct* or *indirect* glans stimulation. With *indirect* stimulation, the structures surrounding the glans are manipulated without actual fingers or hand contact with the glans penis. Women, when masturbating, are less apt to resort to direct touching of their glans (clitoris). This same indirect method of glans stimulation may be used by the intact male, for example, the glans is stimulated by moving the loose skin sheath over the glans. No lubrication is needed.

With *direct* stimulation, the glans is actually touched, with no interpositioning of adjacent parts of the genitals. Some type of extraneous lubrication usually is needed, for example, saliva, KY jelly, creams, oils, lotions, etc.

Obviously, the intact male can stimulate the glans by *either* the direct or indirect method. The circumcised male has no such option. The mobility of his skin sheath has been lost by its shortening and relatively tight attachment to the penile shaft behind the glans. Unwittingly he has been denied some options for sexual dalliance.

But the ingenious male—circumcised or not—will find ways to masturbate!

23. The History of Circumcision Is Filled with Hysteria, Bias, Misinformation, etc.

- *Circumcision represents a subtraction.*
- *Almost every male infant is born with a snug, irrectractable foreskin.*
- *Very few doctors in the United States know how to care for the infant's foreskin.*

A large amount of what is written about circumcision simply is not true. This applies to articles that appear in the lay magazines and in respected scientific journals. Most people do not realize that circumcision represents a subtraction. Physicians who mastered calculus and statistical analysis in pre-med school overlook this simple fact. Urologists have stated that they are not aware that the prepuce has a function. An anatomist states that there is no difference in sensitivity between the circumcised and the intact penis, and quotes as his reference to prove his point a nebulous, invalid experiment by one of our foremost sexologists. Another urologist has no understanding of the function of the frenulum in eliciting sexual pleasure. Most physicians do not know, or do not believe, that almost every infant is born with a snug, irretractable foreskin, and that the foreskin is always attached to the glans at birth. Very, very, very few doctors in the United States know how to care for and wash the foreskin.

An article by a clinical psychologist that appeared in a widely circulated national medical journal devoted to human sexuality stirred my ire. This man was on the faculty of a medical school. His hodge-podge of uninformed, imbecilic drivel included the following: "For the child's well being and optimal development, circumcision was necessary, so that one looked genitally like his peers. Not to circumcise involved taking risks and creating dilemmas where neither need exist. The circumcised penis is cleaner, special, unique, and more cared for, whereas the (normal) penis is inferior, defective and less valued. The uncircumcised child in a circumcised peer group often finds that the only other uncircumcised boy in his school is a refugee, migrant, or minority child—someone from an environment with poor medical standards." It is difficult to be silently complacent in the face of such remarkable nonsense.

Ann Briggs, in her excellent book, *Circumcision: What Every Parent Should Know*, presents a concise history of circumcision. This chapter of her work puts circumcision into historical perspective.[7]

"The precise origins of the procedure we call circumcision are unknown. However, most authorities agree that it did not originate with the Jewish people. It is also fairly certain that it apparently sprang up spontaneously in different areas of the world, as fairly widely scattered groups, with no apparent common ancestor or connecting link, have practiced the procedure. It has been suggested that initially, in primitive tribal societies, it was a way of humiliating and/or outwardly marking those captured into slavery, possibly as a symbolic substitution for the more dangerous castration. Throughout most of recorded history, however, circumcision has been a ritual, establishing a visible sign of a covenant with God. In other societies, largely in Africa and Australia, it was a rite of passage, performed at puberty or prior to marriage.

"Most groups that have traditionally practiced circumcision have been located in the Middle East, Africa, or Asia, with the very center of the practice being the Middle East. In addition, although there are a few notable exceptions, the vast majority of peoples who have circumcised were either Semitic people or those in their direct sphere of influence. Circumcision is a relative newcomer to Europe and North America. Except for Jews living in Europe who, of course, have circumcised throughout their history, no group of people living in Europe in recorded history is known to have practiced the surgery. The same holds true for North America: except for one group of Eskimos, no group in North America practiced circumcision. Temple drawings show that genital mutilations were practiced in South America. It is not known, however, how common the procedure we call circumcision (simply removing the foreskin) was there.

23. (continued)
The History of Circumcision Is Filled with Hysteria, Bias, Misinformation, etc.

- *The origins of the surgery in a medical context are bizarre to a modern reader.*
  Circumcision: What Every Parent Should Know

- *"Some obstetricians have made early circumcision a fetish . . . one instance . . . in which the operation was performed when the [infant male's] hips had been delivered and pending expulsion of the upper half of the body."*
  Diseases of the Newborn,
  A.T. Schaeffer, M.D.

"Throughout history, there are several basic patterns which emerge regarding circumcision practice. First, circumcision is relatively rare when taken against the whole panorama of history. Most societies for most of human history did not circumcise. Currently, between 10% and 20% of the world's male population is circumcised. In other words, throughout the whole of human history, only a minority of men have been circumcised. Second, circumcision has only rarely been an infant ritual. Historically, the Jewish people are the only other major group known to have circumcised infants. In most other situations, it was performed as a rite of passage, either at the beginning or at the end of puberty. Third, in virtually every society throughout history for which we have any documented evidence, circumcision has been imposed by the superior and more powerful on the inferior and the weaker. It has been imposed on captured slaves, children, teenagers and babies. It has almost never been the individual's own choice. Felix Bryk, in his book, *Sex and Circumcision, A Study of Phallic Worship and Mutilation in Men and Women*, provides several illustrations of ritual and tribal circumcision. One photograph shows an African tribal circumcision. In it, a boy of approximately ten to twelve years is being pinned down securely by three adult men. In another illustration, a copy of an Egyptian temple relief, a somewhat younger child (six to eight) is being circumcised by a priest while another priest holds the child's hands behind his back. Even in societies where the ritual was performed as a late-puberty or pre-marriage rite and the individual had some choice, the alternatives were usually quite grim. Usually, the options involved total social rejection, from not being considered a warrior or not being allowed to marry, to being turned out from the tribe altogether.

"All this changed in the 19th century with the beginnings of 'medical' circumcision. The origins of the surgery in a medical context are bizarre to a modern reader. In the 18th century, a sociological phenomenon arose that one researcher has called the 'masturbation mania.' Physicians in several European countries argued that masturbation was not only a sin, but a medical problem which could cause mental and physical disease. It was blamed for a variety of physical and mental ills, among them epilepsy, stammering, acne, blindness, and, the most dread of all, masturbatory insanity. Although these ideas seem ludicrous, even impossible to a modern reader, it is important to remember just how primitive medicine was 175 years ago. The very basic concepts of modern medicine (for example, the idea that infection and many diseases are caused by microbes) were unknown. Bloodletting was still the mainstay of medical practice in the United States and most of Europe. One modern researcher has stated that one of the prevailing medical theories was that 'all disease could be reduced to one basic causal model, either the diminution or decrease of nervous energy.' One of the most obvious manifestations of the release of nervous energy is in sexual activity, i.e., orgasm.

"These ideas led to the rise of a whole (largely American) school of medical thought linking sexuality and disease. One of the basic tenets of this way of thinking was that, if overindulgence in 'normal' sexual practices could result in disease, what must indulgence in abnormal sexual practices cause? Sylvester Graham, inventor of Graham crackers, was a strong supporter of these theories. He wrote a book on the subject which listed dozens of diseases that sexual excesses could cause. According to Graham, even sexual thoughts could cause disease. Fortunately, there was a cure for sexual abuse. According to Graham, one could be helped by eating Graham crackers.

"Slowly, the idea of sexual abuse focused on one issue, masturbation, which, by the 1880s, had become the term applied by some to all 'unnatural' sex, from homosexuality to the use of contraception. Another individual who did a great deal of 'research' in this area was John Harvey Kellogg, whose breakfast cereal company is still well known. According to Kellogg, masturbation could cause no fewer than 31 diseases, among them 'prolapse of the rectum, atrophy of the testes, general exhaustion,' and, of course, insanity. Fortunately, Kellogg made an additional 'discovery.' A masturbator could be identified by the manifestation of one or more of 38 tell-tale signs, among them changes in personality, shyness, poor posture, acne, insomnia, or biting the fingernails. There could hardly have been a child alive at the time (1882) who did not show at least one of these 'significant' symptoms, so it is easy to understand that such thinking caused deep concern among parents. What parent wanted his child to suffer the supposedly terrible consequences of masturbation? Kellogg, like Graham, fortuitously discovered a help for masturbators: they could be cured by eating Kellogg's breakfast cereals! In addition to this nutritional solution, however, Kellogg suggested another possible cure for adolescent boys who persisted in the practice: circumcision without anesthesia.

"It would be merely curious history if the writings of Graham and Kellogg could be dismissed as a bizarre, short-lived set of attitudes towards sexuality. However, although neither of these men was a physician, they were prominent, rich industrialists (in a society that followed rich industrialists with nearly the interest that today is given to prominent movie stars), and their works were widely read and believed by lay people and by physicians. The physicians, while sharing the lay writers' horror of masturbation, totally abandoned any suggestion of nutritional cures, and advocated only the totally medical cure: circumcision. However, the physicians took the reasoning one step further. Instead of performing circumcision on those already indulging in sexual abuses (in other words, using circumcision as a *cure*), it was suggested that circumcision be performed on every child in infancy as a *preventive measure*. The reasoning was that the foreskin needed to be retracted for cleaning and drew the child's attention to his penis, causing masturbation. The simple solution? If the foreskin were removed, the child would not need to 'think' about his penis, and therefore would not masturbate.

"One writer has suggested that the rise of circumcision as a cure for masturbation was a combined attempt of parents and physicians to control a child's sexuality during a period of history (the industrial revolution) in which there was beginning to be a great deal of instability in the family. Karen Paige says: 'Masturbation frightened middle class parents because doctors said it explained why so many young people were neurotic, disobedient, disrespectful of parental authority, and oversexed . . . I suspect that circumcision solved some of the dilemmas confronting both the middle class families and the newly established (and not yet entirely respectable) obstetrical and surgical professions. Parents wanted to control the sexual impulses of their children; physicians wanted to demonstrate and consolidate their new powers.'

"By the late 1800s, medical ideas began to change. While it was still believed that masturbation was harmful and that circumcision could prevent masturbation, the idea that masturbation could cause insanity and diseases like epilepsy was losing hold. Circumcisions in Great Britain began declining, but at this point, medical thinking in the United States took an even more bizarre twist. As incredibly as it sounds, some doctors began attributing medical problems to the presence of foreskin *in and of itself*. Formerly, it was believed that the presence of a foreskin contributed to masturbation and that masturbation caused these diseases. However, the belief changed in such a way that masturbation was dropped out of the cycle, and the foreskin supposedly caused the diseases directly. Theoretically, then, circumcision, *simply by removing the foreskin*, could cure or prevent problems such as alcoholism, epilepsy, plague, paralysis, rheumatism, polio, lunacy, tuberculosis, syphilis, and many other diseases and conditions. Of course, acceptance of these ideas only reinforced the thinking that neonatal circumcision, as a preventive measure, made really good medical sense.

"In 1891, a book on circumcision appeared entitled *History of Circumcision From the Earliest Times to the Present*. Written by a physician, Peter Remondino, the book is incredible, containing the most unscientific statements and medical errors imaginable. Remondino states that circumcision

---

23. *(continued)*
The History of Circumcision Is Filled with Hysteria, Bias, Misinformation, etc.

■ *Theoretically, then, circumcision, simply by removing the foreskin, could cure or prevent problems such as alcoholism, epilepsy, plague, paralysis, rheumatism, polio, lunacy, tuberculosis, syphilis, and many other diseases and conditions.*

Circumcision: What Every Parent Should Know

23. (continued)
The History of Circumcision Is Filled with Hysteria, Bias, Misinformation, etc.

■ *Instead of slowly abandoning the idea of circumcision, however, the American medical community simply adopted other rationales.*
Circumcision: What Every Parent Should Know

■ *In America, during the past 100 years or so, circumcision has had a strong irrational bias that has been constantly seeking validation.*
Marilyn Milos, R.N.

can cure or prevent nearly 100 different conditions. He suggests that there is a relationship between foreskin length and intelligence. And even though this is supposedly a book on circumcision for physicians, he digresses to comment on such diverse subjects as female appearance by international region and the Germans as a superior race. It would be nice to be able to dismiss this work as a medical and historical curiosity, but the fact is that this book was very popular with the medical community of the time and played a very significant role in increasing the acceptance of the operation within the American medical community. The book has, in fact, been reprinted many times (the latest in 1974) and is still available today. Edward Wallerstein reports that as of 1983, Remondino's book was still listed in the New York City Public Library catalog, and that the catalog listed the republication date (1974), making no reference to the fact that this was merely a republication of a work that was over 80 years old.

"Circumcision became the 'wonder drug' of 19th century American medicine. Some writers of this era even began recommending circumcision of the clitoris so that females could reap the same health benefits. The pinnacle of this thinking is perhaps an article published in the *Journal of the American Medical Association* in 1910 which touts a new circumcision clamp, one so easy to use that 'a person could circumcise himself, provided that he did not become faint-hearted.'

"Slowly, medical thinking did change. Partly, one must assume, the change in attitudes occurred simply because physicians started to see their theories disproved in practice. Circumcised men got epilepsy. Circumcised men became alcoholics. Circumcised men got tuberculosis, rheumatism, and went insane. *Clearly, it became obvious that circumcision was not preventing anything, even masturbation.* Instead of slowly abandoning the idea of circumcision, however, the *American medical community simply adopted other rationales.* Beginning in the 1930's, some physicians began insisting that circumcision would prevent cancer of the penis and the prostate, and in the spouses of circumcised men, cancer of the cervix.

"In the late 1940s, an additional rationale arose. Based on the number of young men who 'needed' to be circumcised during World War II conscription, the idea that 'he might need it later' was repeated. At the same time, the idea that circumcision could prevent venereal disease, which had existed since the 1800s, gained new credibility as research which seemed to support this idea was reviewed in *Newsweek*. And in the 1950s, parents' magazines and baby books began advocating circumcision as necessary for social acceptance and as beneficial for reasons of cleanliness, the constant implication being that the uncircumcised penis was quite difficult to clean and that infections were common among uncircumcised boys and men."

"In America, during the past 100 years or so, circumcision has had a strong irrational bias that has been constantly seeking validation. Our medical community has used one reason after another to justify a surgery that most of the modern world has never even considered," says Marilyn Milos of NOCIRC, and who could disagree.

Victims' Voices . . .

"One unique argument for circumcision in English-speaking countries—now rejected in all English-speaking nations except the U.S.—is the notion that circumcision has a 'prophylactic' value, that it 'prevents' certain problems from developing. As a surgery, the concept is a bizarre one, now applied solely to the genitals. No other body part is subject to 'routine' removal as a 'preventive' measure, especially when measured against the pain and risks of surgery. A review and rebuttal of all the silly claims made by pro-circumcisers have been done extensively by others. Suffice it to say, if all the claims were true, America's circumcised males would be free of alcoholism, epilepsy, mental illness, venereal disease, cancer, AIDS, and a host of infections, while our intact males would be dead or too sick to get out of bed."

Marilyn Milos,
R.N., NOCIRC

24. Christianity Does Not Require or Promote Circumcision

The God-man Christ was a Jew and a teacher. His Jewish parents, Mary and Joseph, conformed to the theological dictates of the Jewish religion, and accordingly, Christ was circumcised. But this act of obedient conformity did not require subsequent followers of Christ—the Christians—to be circumcised. This issue of circumcision was addressed shortly after the death of Christ by St. Paul: "For in Jesus Christ neither circumcision availeth anything, nor uncircumcision, but faith which worketh by love (St. Paul to the Galatians)."

According to St. Paul, "Spirituality and Christian love are not found in an operation, a cutting of a part of the body, but in the inspiration, caring, and love that exist in one's heart. Therefore, the operation is meaningless in regards to whether or not one is a follower of Christ."

To the best of my knowledge, the position of all Christian religions in regard to circumcision remains unchanged from that of St. Paul.

In the last decade or so, an interesting change occurred in the name of one of the Catholic Church's Holy Days: January 1st was formerly "The Feast of the Circumcision," but now the name has been changed to "Mary, Mother of God." I do not know what prompted the change. Possibly, many church members had thoughts and opinions similar to my mother's: "There is no logic in sanctifying the destruction of a normal structure that God had just created."

It is inconceivable that the myriad complex biological systems existing in our universe have come into being by pure chance, by a repetitive throw of the evolutionary dice. There must be a God! One instinctively and logically knows that an object as simple as a tea cup, for example, could never "be," as a result of fortuitous physical-chemical combinations. An intelligent force, man, must be behind its creation.

How less likely it is that the infinitely more complex man would evolve by mere chance from random mutations. Logically, I concede the existence of a Supreme Creator—God!

God then bequeaths us our normal bodies. When a child is born, everyone wishes most ardently that the infant be normal in every way. Yet here in the United States, within a day or so of the birth of our male children, we deliberately surgically, permanently alter the genitals. Is this done out of ignorance, or ingratitude, or out of blatant arrogance? Would any of us wish that the child have less than normal sight, or hearing, or smell? The surgical act seems incongruous and at variance to the gratitude and kindness we should have in our hearts at the birth of a normal child.

There was much discussion of some Christians' "endorsement" of infant male circumcision at the 2nd International Symposium on Circumcision held in 1991. Here are the highlights[8]. "Christianity largely ignored the subject of physical circumcision of the male for nearly 2,000 years. During those centuries, the Old Testament era was viewed by theologians and laymen alike as a symbolic preparation for the life and work of Jesus Christ, and Old Testament law as symbolic depictions of the sacrifice He was to make for the salvation of mankind. Then, just about at the turn of this century, a very interesting phenomenon took place. Modern medicine began to come of age! The role of the doctor, as well as that of the entire field of medicine, changed dramatically. The priest and the minister rather suddenly found themselves competing with the doctor in terms of giving advice and counsel in matters of health and even life-style. It does not seem overly unkind to note that modern medicine at that point in its history began to take on a rather God-like aura, certainly where issues of life and death were concerned. Nowhere within the broad scope of the 20th-century medicine is its power and influence more apparent than in the field of preventive medicine. Diseases which were seen at one time as most likely terminal, and often as an act of

- *God bequeathed us our normal body. Should we alter it out of ignorance, ingratitude, or blatant arrogance?*

- *Who of us would wish that our child would have less than a normal body?*

- *"No one . . . should circumcise himself or his son for any reason but pure faith."*
  Rabbi Moses Maimonides

24. (continued)
Christianity Does Not Require or Promote Circumcision

- *People function best with their complete normal faculties—hearing, sight, smell, etc. Love and sexual function between a man and a woman are served best by the normal genitals with which they are endowed at birth. Who presumes to improve upon that which is normal?*

God, were re-examined in light of new discoveries and rendered both treatable and preventable. It was, therefore, to modern medicine that Americans increasingly looked for relief from their suffering and cures for their diseases. Unfortunately, for the American male, preventive medicine early in this century incorporated the practice of infant male circumcision. This fact is especially unfortunate because it set off a counter-reaction within large segments of the Christian community.

"No one should minimize the reaction of Christianity in America to the medical field's claims for routine infant male circumcision as a preventive health measure. That reaction not only helped to establish and legitimize the procedure but has worked to retain it long after claims of medical benefit have been successfully challenged and the practice set aside by the rest of the industrialized world. The overwhelming reaction among American Christians, not unlike that of some Jews, was a rather smug, 'We told you so! Our God has always been right. You just think that you discovered a good thing. We've known about it for centuries.' It was indeed a kind of 'anything you can do, our God has always done better,' or, at the very least, 'our God said it long before you did!' The medical profession was simply not going to be allowed to upstage God!

"For the first time in 2,000 years, some Christians began to look with new eyes at Old Testament teachings. If infant male circumcision was the right thing to do, what about the other Old Testament laws? The claim that the Old Testament contains medical prescriptions in ritual form has been disputed among Jews for centuries. Most Orthodox Jews have rejected such claims out of hand, particularly where circumcision, the 'seal of the covenant,' is concerned. In the words of Moses Maimonides (1135-1204): 'No one... should circumcise himself or his son for any other reason but pure faith.' Other Jewish writers, however, including Josephus in the 1st century, have insisted that circumcision has both hygienic and medical benefits.

"Christians claiming health benefits for male circumcision as prescribed by Old Testament law is, on the other hand, a much newer phenomenon. While it seems clear that these Christian claims have come about largely as a reaction to the growing dominance and authority of 20th-century medicine, such attitudes and claims have become common throughout modern-day Christianity.

"It has been suggested by some Christians (and some Jews) that circumcision is just one more of the means by which God provided hygienic protection for his children, particularly during their desert wanderings. What many Christians do not realize, however, is that Israel did not circumcise her male infants during her 40-year wanderings in the Wilderness (Joshua 5: 4 & 5). When this fact is looked at, together with the effects of God's judgment upon the unbelieving congregation of Israel, a very interesting fact emerges. Remember, as a judgment, God detained Israel in the Wilderness until the last of those who had come out of Egypt had died, except the two faithful spies. This means, then, that the males who were circumcised just as they entered the Promised Land were up to 40 years of age and were fathers and even grandfathers at the time of their circumcision.

"If, as some suggest, God conceived infant male circumcision as a protective health measure, doesn't it seem rather strange that he risked not only the health of the individual males born in the Wilderness but the very propagation of the new generations who were to claim the Promised Land? In light of all the stringent requirements God imposed upon Israel in the Wilderness and all the lessons of obedience he taught them, why would He have allowed virtually every male in the congregation of Israel to remain uncircumcised until they arrived at the very border of the new land? Was their circumcision as they crossed over the Jordan into the Promised Land a matter of health or symbolic holiness?

"The Scriptural evidence clearly will not support the idea of Old Testament circumcision as a health measure. Neither the then-practiced style of circumcision nor the periods when God condoned noncompliance suggest any such interpretation.

"A similar conclusion seems justified for all Old Testament ordinances. In 1963, Dr. S.I. McMillen published his best-selling book, *None of These Diseases,* in which he maintains that the Old Testament contains God's medical prescriptions for human diseases. The unbiased reader is struck, however, by how carefully Old Testament examples seem to be selected and even redefined. The order to cast out lepers to live alone outside the camp is explained by God: '. . . that they may not defile their camp, in the midst of which I dwell.' And the Scriptures go on to say, 'And the people of Israel did so, and drove them outside the camp . . . ' (Numbers 5: 3 & 4 RSV). That event is defined by Dr. McMillen as 'quarantine.' Further, he does not even mention the shunning of women during menses. One can only imagine the psychological toll that such regular rejection would take on women. Clearly, many Old Testament laws have an element of sacrifice in them. Logically, you cannot pick and choose at will. Old Testament law handed down by an all-wise God is either *all* good medicine or it is *all* something else! In looking over just the more common laws, it seems quite justifiable to conclude that God's intent and purpose was not to reveal medical knowledge in the law but to fashion a unique people upon the earth! Jewish laws and traditions are best understood as religious observances in terms of the 'seal of the covenant' and symbolic purity and sacrifice."

Christians may also want to read Chapter 25 carefully. It reveals that Old Testament circumcision, practiced by Jews century after century until after the New Testament era, involved only cutting off the tip of the foreskin!

24. *(continued)* Christianity Does Not Require or Promote Circumcision

- *Old Testament circumcision, practiced by the Jews century after century, involved only cutting off the tip of the foreskin, and not the entire foreskin.*

25. Some Jews Are Even Changing Their Minds About Circumcision

- *Would God's covenant be fulfilled by a more humane religious ceremony?*

Circumcision, for the Jews, is strictly a religious act. It is in keeping with their covenant with God: By fulfilling the Commandment of Circumcision, every person has an opportunity to bring a sacrifice to the Almighty.

"This is my covenant which ye shall keep, between me and you and thy seed after thee: every man-child among you shall be circumcised (Genesis 17:10)." "And the uncircumcised man whose flesh of his foreskin is not circumcised, that soul shall be cut off from his people. He hath broken my covenant (Genesis 17:14)."

The Jews then have a belief, a covenant with God, an act of faith—all reasons associated with their religion—for performing circumcision. They make no claim that it is done for hygiene reasons, to forestall masturbation, or to lessen the incidence of cancer of the penis or cervix.

Brith (bris) milah is a most sacred religious ceremony. Its whole purpose *is not medical* and there is a vast difference between the normal medical approach and the requirements of brith milah. Thus, Jewish religious requirements are not met by secular surgical circumcision.

The circumcision technique of Orthodox Jews differs from modern clamping techniques. Rabbinical authorities in Jerusalem and throughout the world have asserted that "the use of clamping instruments that prevent bleeding during the circumcision is not in accordance with Jewish Religious Law." After the mohel (the rabbi or representative performing the circumcision) removes the outer skin segment of the prepuce with a cutting instrument, he now tears the remaining mucous membrane portion of the foreskin off all around the corona of the glans by taking hold of the flaps of the foreskin with his thumb and forefinger. Every vestige of the foreskin is destroyed. According to Jewish law, "The tender covering under the skin is to be rent with the fingernails. Circumcision without tearing is equivalent to no circumcision at all."

Rabbi Moses Maimonides, the revered theologian and philosopher, summed this up in the 13th century: "No one should circumcise himself or his son for any reason but pure faith . . ." But the physical act of cutting the sensitive penis places the Jew on the horns of a dilemma. On the one hand, he is honored to be singled out by God for the covenant of circumcision. But as a compassionate human being, he abhors the pain inflicted upon his beloved infant. And make no mistake. Cutting off the foreskin hurts!

Alternate brith ceremonies that would be less painful have been considered. One is aware that today most reform and conservative mohels have abandoned the older technique—whereby the inner layer of the adherent foreskin is torn with the mohel's fingernails—believing that the modern clamping devices are safer and more humane. And circumcising the infant on the eighth post natal day is not always adhered to. Concessions then have already been made to the stricter, older ceremonial stipulations.

Let us engage in a semantic digression, for the moment, for a possible solution to the Jew's dilemma. *Webster's New International Dictionary*, 2nd Edition, and Dorland's *The American Illustrated Medical Dictionary*, 9th Edition, may provide some assistance. Both dictionaries define circumcision as "a cutting around" (as the bark of a tree). On the other hand, "ectomy" is defined as the "excision of or the removal of" an object (e.g. an appendectomy is the removal of the appendix; a mastectomy is the removal of the breasts, etc.). The removal of the foreskin (or prepuce) then would be a "prepucectomy."

How did the term circumcision expand to include the radical excision of the foreskin when what the word circumcision implies is a much less radical procedure of merely making a simple, superficial encircling cut of the penis that does no significant damage to the end of the penis? God's covenant would be fulfilled by this more humane ceremony. Even a local anesthesia with a fine number 30 gauge needle could be used.

Ironically, the historic record demonstrates that the original circumcision practiced by the Jews was quite moderate compared to either modern Jewish or "medical" circumcision. The history of circumcision was presented and discussed at the 2nd International Symposium on Circumcision held in 1991. Here is a summary of the findings[9].

"The Scriptures state simply that God told Abraham to circumcise himself and all of his offspring and slaves who were eight days of age or older. And, on the `selfsame day,' Abraham did it. The act which Abraham performed was, in fact, milah—the symbolic removal of the tip of the foreskin. This relatively simple form of circumcision was practiced by the Jews for approximately 2,000 years, throughout the whole of the Old (and, for that matter, the New) Testament era. No other feature was added to the rite until sometime around 140 A.D.

"The foreskin and the glans are typically fused together at birth and are actually a single organ at that stage of development. Therefore, when the ancient circumciser simply cut off the protruding tip of the typical infant foreskin with a single cut, a great deal of the natural foreskin would have been left intact. Such a penis would have continued to go through its natural developmental stages. That is, the remaining foreskin would have separated naturally over time from the glans. This process would have left the glans with many of its natural features—texture, sensitivity, etc. Such a penis would also have had a rather ample remnant of foreskin. And, since the frenulum would not have been directly or intentionally destroyed, the foreskin remnant would most likely have stayed in place and continued to cover a substantial portion of the glans. It is, indeed, this very fact which allowed `renegade' Jews for nearly 2,000 years to effect a rather simple and convincing foreskin restoration, or re-covering of the glans.

"It wasn't until after the time of Christ that Periah was introduced. Periah is the second step or procedure in ritual circumcision. After cutting off the end of the infant foreskin, periah consists of tearing and stripping back the remaining inner lining of the foreskin off the glans and then, by the use of a sharpened fingernail, removing all such mucous tissue including the excising of the frenulum.

"Jewish historians differ as to exactly when this second step was introduced into ritual circumcision. Few historians, however, disagree as to *why* it was introduced: circumcision without it was simply too easily disguised! Quite simply, rabbis sought to put an end once and for all to Jews passing themselves off as uncircumcised males by enlongating the remainder of their foreskin. The rabbis' solution was to so entirely obliterate the foreskin that any Jew so circumcised would not be able to disguise `the seal of the covenant.'

"It is interesting to note, from a historical point of view, that, according to the date, 140 A.D., given in the *Jewish Encyclopedia* for the Institution of Periah, all Biblical Jews—both Old and New Testament—would have been circumcised in the less radical, symbolic style of milah. This being the case, *no* biblical reference to circumcision *ever* refers to or indicates the more radical style of circumcision which is now practiced by modern-day Jews or by the American medical profession.

"There has been an ongoing, and sometimes humorous, debate over why Michelangelo's very famous statue of David has a foreskin. Surely a man with Michelangelo's knowledge of the male anatomy and of history would have known not to put a foreskin on a Jewish youth. Was he simply too embarrassed to chisel the more intimate details of the denuded glans? Did he consider the circumcised penis unaesthetic? Were all his models uncircumcised, and he blindly sculpted what he saw? These, and other speculations, have been raised in an effort to solve this mystery chiseled in stone.

"More recently, as greater knowledge has been gained regarding circumcision practices throughout history,

---

25. *(continued)*
Some Jews Are Even Changing Their Minds About Circumcision

- *"Will the liberal rabbinate, in view of the impending changes in the medical approach to nonreligious circumcision, also suggest changes in the Jewish ritual? Let us hope that sanity, not hysteria, will prevail in approaching this potentially vexing problem."*
Edward Wallerstein, Circumcision and Anti-Semitism: An Update. *Humanistic Judaism*, Winter 1983.

25. (continued)
Some Jews Are Even Changing Their Minds About Circumcision

- *Old Testament circumcision, practiced by the Jews century after century, involved only cutting off the tip of the foreskin, and not the entire foreskin.*

- *Also during New Testament time, bris milah (cutting off only the tip) was practiced.*

Editor's Note...

The purpose of this chapter is not to impugn the Jewish rite of circumcision, but only to present some of the issues being discussed in the Jewish community.

---

other explanations have been offered. Recently, a most compelling theory has been put forward by Edward Wallerstein. After discussing some of the possible explanations noted above, he states, 'However, there is another solution and I believe I have found it. Michelangelo probably knew exactly what he was doing. First, it is necessary to examine the precise method of circumcision in 1000 B.C. [around the time of David's birth]. Originally the procedure called for removing *only* the very tip of the foreskin. Known in Hebrew as milah ... The glans of David's penis is almost completely covered by the foreskin. This factor probably prompted physicians to claim that Michelangelo sculpted the penis as uncircumcised. However, the tip of the foreskin—the preputial orifice which, normally covers the meatus (urinary opening) and usually extends beyond the glans—is ablated [removed] ... In addition, the sculpting of this statue was not a hasty affair. Michelangelo labored on it for four years. We can assume that with his astute knowledge of anatomy he was as meticulous in penile details as in all others. It is therefore probable that Michelangelo correctly portrayed David as circumcised, based upon the surgical procedure of that period—that is, with only the very tip of the foreskin removed.'

"Whether or not Wallerstein's theory about the statue of David is correct, the fact remains that a male who had only the tip of his infant foreskin removed would have retained a rather goodly portion of his natural foreskin. Such a penis, when flaccid, might well appear to our American-trained eyes to be uncircumcised.

"There is no contention here that Jewish doctors are responsible for introducing or promoting infant circumcision as a medical practice in the United States. There is, however, an apparent procedural link between Judaism and routine medical circumcision. Of all the peoples on earth who ritualistically circumcise their young males, Judaism is the only major group which performs the rite in infancy. Early in this century, when routine male circumcision was believed to prevent an array of potentially dangerous conditions, it was also believed that infants do not feel pain in the first few days of life. Therefore, it was the *routine circumcision of the infant male* which the American medical profession eventually espoused.

"There seems little doubt that members of the medical community in this country turned for advice and example to those practitioners with the most knowledge and experience. It was, after all, Jewish mohels who had centuries of tradition and experience—including being called upon to circumcise such dignitaries as the English royal family, etc. The most striking consequence of this rather obvious cross-pollination is the fact that the style of current medical circumcision closely resembles the results of Jewish ritual circumcision. In both instances the glans penis is completely bared and little or no excess skin is left on the shaft of the penis. This fact is noteworthy, since most medical journals and practitioners in this country would maintain that the purpose of routine medical circumcision is simply to prevent phimoses and to accommodate hygiene. The complete denuding of the glans and the removal of virtually all mobile skin on the penile shaft are clearly not necessary to accomplish these stated purposes. It is far more likely that both the definition and the style of infant circumcision were `borrowed from the experts' by the relatively inexperienced medical profession around the turn of this century."

So we see that originally and for centuries, Jewish circumcision was similar to the minor procedure that was suggested earlier in this chapter. Could Jews someday return to the removal of the very tip of the foreskin?

A re-examination of circumcision (brit milah) is occurring within the Jewish community itself.[10] A sampling of Jewish writings of the last decade illustrate this process: •"A Mother Questions Brit Milah" •"Letter to Our Son's Grandparents: Why We Decided Against Circumcision"•"A Baby-Naming Ceremony, Rochester Society for Humanistic Judaism" • "Jesse's Circumcision."

26. Don't Be Fooled, Most Books, Including Medical Text Books, Contain Inaccurate Information

It is amazing how much improper advice is given to parents by American physicians on the false premise that neonatal foreskin attachment and non-retractability are abnormalities that must be corrected by circumcision. Many texts refer to this condition as phimosis, but it isn't. An adherence of the foreskin is normal in infants. True phimosis is the inability to retract the foreskin after puberty.

Below are several examples of misinformation that appear in medical texts relating to the issue of circumcision and "phimosis":

1. "Circumcision: The surgical removal of the prepuce of the penis. Done for hygienic reasons. The foreskin is often tight after birth. It should be pulled back gently at birth to see that the meatus is clear, and then left alone for eight days. After this, if it is tight, it should be picked up in the thumb and finger and gently coaxed backwards twice a day. If it is inclined to bleed, smear it with an antibiotic ointment. Care must be taken not to strip it backwards too far or constriction of the glans (paraphimosis) may occur. If tightness still persists or there is any difficulty in passing urine, a doctor should be consulted. Often the gentle passage of a probe by a doctor, underneath the skin of the prepuce, will obviate any need to circumcise." (Taber's *Cyclopedic Medical Dictionary*, 13th Edition)

   Using these criteria, every male would qualify for a circumcision.

2. "Circumcision is a simple innocuous procedure but it can, and too often is, done incorrectly. The most common congenital malformation of the penis is phimosis. The name is properly applied only to those cases in which the preputial orifice is so small that retraction of the prepuce is difficult or impossible. Phimosis is treated by circumcision or posthectomy, which consists of the removal of a part of the prepuce, including the narrow preputial orifice." (*Plastic and Reconstructive Surgery*, Hans May, Third Edition)

   Using these criteria, every male would qualify for a circumcision.

3. "Circumcision, if indicated, is usually performed within the first few days of life . . . circumcision is usually requested by the parents and is rarely medically indicated; however, if the foreskin is tight and cannot be retracted, circumcision is required." (*The Merck Manual*, 13th Edition)

   Using these criteria, every male would qualify for a circumcision.

But a glint of truth and sunshine appear in the 14th Edition of the *Merck Manual*. It succinctly states: "Circumcision is rarely medically indicated."

Browsing through your neighborhood bookstore seeking advice on the care of the normal intact infant's penis can be a confusing, painstaking experience. The amount of **poor advice** given is boundless:

- "Pull the foreskin back so as to see the urethral opening."
- "Circumcision promotes cleanliness."
- "Circumcision is necessary so as to look genitally like one's peers."
- "Circumcision is required if retraction is not possible."
- "One must massage, retract, knead, stretch the foreskin."

But progress is being made. As you see on the back cover of this book and in Chapter 38, Dr. Benjamin Spock, the most noted child care author, has reversed his opinion on circumcision, and now opposes it.

- *Leave it alone!*

27. Don't Accept, at Face Value, What Your Doctor Has to Say About Circumcision

- *Physicians can clearly influence the circumcision rates at their hospitals by their attitude towards circumcision and their willingness or unwillingness to educate parents.*

- *"Most parents want the operation. I can make an extra $200. Why should I try to dissuade them?"*

    Obstetrician

- *"If I don't do it, the pediatrician will, and he'll get the money."*

    Obstetrician/Gynecologist

There was a time when I discussed the merit, or lack of merit, of neonatal circumcision with various physicians in our hospital. My principal argument against neonatal circumcision is the obvious lack of an indication for removing a normal structure. My discussions with the obstetricians were enlightening. One told me that most parents wanted the procedure. He could realize an extra $200 on the operation; he saw no reason, therefore, to dissuade them. Another told me that if he did not do the circumcision, the pediatricians or someone else would do it, and make the extra money. Another physician thought it was too tedious and time consuming to tell the mother how to clean and care for the normal penis. It was much simpler to merely remove the foreskin.

On one occasion when the parent did not have her son circumcised but returned to the obstetrician's office about a month later to ask his advice about her son's reddened foreskin, the doctor suggested and then performed a circumcision. He mildly upbraided the mother for not having the operation done initially, as he had suggested. The doctor, obviously, failed completely in understanding the problem: it was far better that the less sensitive, less important protective foreskin get reddened from an ammonia-laden diaper than to have the delicate glans irritated. The obstetrician should have known that from the moment of circumcision, the exposed *glans* would forever bear the brunt of contact with urine, feces, wet diapers, and clothing. The reddened foreskin was a sign telling him one of the important functions of the foreskin. He completely missed the message.

Another physician, a urologist, gave me a most remarkable reason why he favored routine circumcision. In all sincerity he claimed that in the Orient, over 18% of males develop penile cancer (an invalid claim). He advanced this argument to justify the circumcision of all male babies in the state of Pennsylvania. He also remarked that the obtunding (dulling) of glans sensation would result in less frequent premature ejaculation. He made no mention of how he thought this obtundation might affect males at the other, older end of the life span in regards to impotence. He failed also in observing that the incidence of premature ejaculation is just as great in circumcised males as in the intact.

Discussing the pros and cons with the nurses was another consideration. Some nurses sensibly could sift cold logic from myths and prejudices. One politely listened and then had her baby circumcised anyway. I had the impression that her husband felt uncomfortable, and possibly jealous of a child who might have a penis that differed in appearance from him. Many nurses seem unimaginative. I soon gave up on them. Many nurses equate foreskins with old men. This brings us to medical school training. Even with all the emphasis and talk of sex today, medical schools have de-emphasized or even excluded sexual medicine class preferring to put priority on technological medical advances. Thousands of graduating physicians will, therefore, have to be self-taught or otherwise remain as uninformed as the lay person regarding the sexual implications of child rearing, illness, and prescribed treatments. Unresolved sexual problems may have tragic consequences.

Sexuality is an integral part of the total person affecting the way each individual, from birth to death, relates to self, to his or her special partner, and to every other person.

A small but growing number of physicians refuse to perform circumcisions except when medically indicated. And a few hospitals, like Harris County Hospital near Houston and the famous Johns Hopkins Hospital in Baltimore, will no longer allow their facilities to be used for non-medical circumcisions.[7]

Physicians can clearly influence the circumcision rates at their hospitals by their attitude towards circumcision and their willingness or unwillingness to educate parents.

A comprehensive investigation of circumcision in Vermont reported recently in the Burlington Free Press (March 6, 1988) underscored the important role of the doctor. Gifford Memorial Hospital, which pioneered Vermont's first birthing center, refuses to market circumcision and will not circumcise in the first 24 hours of life. Parents are told to take their time in making an important decision for another human being. The consequence is the state's lowest circumcision rate of only 4.0%.

In contrast, at Northwestern Hospital, a pro-circumcision doctor tells parents that his own sons are circumcised and he wouldn't "run the risk" of being intact. That hospital has a circumcision rate of 87.7%, well above the national average of 59% and the state average of 63%.

In my reading, and in discussions with men who are circumcised, I have encountered an almost universal phenomenon: the need of the circumcised male to constantly prove to himself that his surgically altered penis is as sensitive and as functional as the normal penis. (Since the male ego is so closely allied with his genitals, this concern is understandable.)

The nationally known sexologist, William Masters, M.D., attempts to allay this concern by devising a most improbable, unscientific experiment:

> "A limited number of the male study-subject population was exposed to a brief clinical experiment designed to disprove the false premise of excessive sensitivity of the circumcised glans. The 35 uncircumcised males were matched at random with circumcised study subjects of similar ages. Routine neurologic testing for both exteroceptive and light tactile discrimination were conducted on the ventral and dorsal surfaces of the penile body, with particular attention directed toward the glans. No clinically significant difference could be established between the circumcised and the uncircumcised glans during these examinations."

It is almost impossible to speak with any staunch pro-circumcisionist without this experiment and its conclusions being brought into the discussion. A long time ago, I learned to question "the authorities," when what they say is contrary to common sense and reason. My criticisms of Masters' contrived experiment are many:

1. There is obvious prejudice in his subject selection. The volunteers were sought from relatively unrepresentative social, intellectual, and economic backgrounds.

2. The study results were dependent upon subjective interpretation of patients under highly charged emotional and experimental conditions. The artificial atmosphere of a research laboratory might alter psychologic and physiologic patterns and responses.

3. The study fails to mention whether the neurologic testing was conducted with the genitals in a flaccid or turgid state—this would have significant bearing upon the sensory perceptive responses.

4. The type of neurologic testing and stimuli may not have been appropriate.

5. A physician performing a circumcision on an adult always is impressed by the reddened, moist glans that is supersensitive after the anesthesia "wears off." The adult male can now express his feelings and complains about the hypersensitivity. Often the glans must now be protected with cotton, for example, for several weeks until it "toughens up" from its contact with clothing. The male circumcised as an infant has no such complaints, as his glans has been rubbed, abraded, and toughened for years by its contact with a host of extraneous agents.

Masters would be more credible if he had desisted in his effort to prove that "circumcision makes no difference."

27. *(continued)*
Don't Accept, at Face Value, What Your Doctor Has to Say About Circumcision

■ *I have encountered an almost universal phenomenon: the need of the circumcised male to constantly prove to himself that his surgically altered penis is as sensitive and as functional as the normal penis.*

28. Most Physicians Are Circumcised Males, or Female Doctors Whose Husbands/Sons Are Circumcised

- *There is a segment of physicians who are embarrassed by their own circumcision and who have the psychic compulsion to circumcise so that they themselves do not feel genitally inferior or different.*

- *Most physicians are uncomfortable discussing sexual matters.*

- *"The worst thing about circumcision is that it produces circumcisers."*

   John A. Erickson

- *Schadenfroh—"gloating over other people's misfortunes."*

   German adjective

- *"Then is it not also true, that no physician, in so far as he is a physician, considers or enjoins what is for the physician's interest, but that all seek the good of their patients?"*

   Dialogue in Plato's Republic

Over the years, I have become aware of, and thoroughly annoyed at the intrigue, deceit, and ignorance of a large segment of the medical profession who have espoused the merits of routine neonatal circumcision of the American male infant. In many instances the attitude has been engendered by a genuine lack of knowledge of basic genital anatomy and/or physiology. In other instances there has been an unwillingness to coldly and unemotionally confront the basic facts. There has been a financial incentive in some instances. There is sometimes a 'dog in the manger' personal quirk in a segment of physicians who are embarrassed by their own circumcision and who have a psychic compulsion to circumcise so that they themselves do not feel genitally inferior or different.

I now know that most physicians are uncomfortable discussing sexual matters, not only with patients, but also with other physicians. Often any attempt at a serious discussion is met with an inappropriate remark, a smirk, and an end to the discussion. Many doctors have not made peace with their own sexual feelings or have not been honest in their evaluation of their sexual prejudices. Many physicians—and this is especially true of those under the age of 50 or 55, most of whom are circumcised—are advising parents regarding circumcision from their own (doctor's) baseline of less than complete penile function and sensitivity.

Victims' Voices . . .

"At work I have given literature to fellow employees who were expecting. One woman already has a son who was circumcised. Her comment was, "I didn't know they hurt my son that way!" She went on to tell me that the doctor discussed the entire delivery process with her for 10 minutes and said nothing about circumcision except asking her yes or no. Personally, I have raised people's awareness, and infants will be spared because of my efforts.

Personally, I'm not doing too well emotionally. The rage, grief and resentment is not much different from what rape victims have. Fortunately, I have a person who is able to counsel me. It is beyond my understanding at this moment how any society could ever practice such a thing on a mass scale. Circumcision is both child abuse and rape. Those who practice it belong behind bars, not behind a mask of medical acceptability!"

   L.R., Indiana

"I don't think that I am the only man to ever have his urethra severed just behind the head of his penis by an inexperienced intern performing a circumcision. I did not need circumcision. I was 24 years old. The Master Surgeon said, "It is a simple operation, and since you are in the hospital, you might as well have it done . . . I will perform the operation myself."

   K.E., North Carolina

"I was circumcised on my parent's kitchen table when I was three months old. I was premature. My mother never forgot the experience or forgave the doctor."

   L.K., San Jose

29. Make No Mistake, There Is Money in Circumcision

Neonatal circumcision of the male is one of the most frequently performed operations in the United States. About 1.2 million male infants are circumcised each year. Since this operation has been done almost routinely for at least 50 years, possibly as many as 50 million American males lack a foreskin. Probably 70% to 80% of all American males under the age of 50 have been circumcised since birth. This includes physicians.

If over this 50-year period one conservatively assumes an average physician's fee of just $25 per operation, the total cost of circumcision—not including hospital charges nor the cost of treatment of complications—would be about $1.25 billion. The actual physician fee for a single neonatal circumcision in 1993 is between $100 and $250. Country-wide then, doctors are collecting as much as $240 million yearly to perform 1.2 million needless operations upon 1.2 million normal penises.

The year 1984 marked the initiation of governmental mandated cost containment. By eliminating routine circumcision, a procedure already deemed superfluous by the American Academy of Pediatrics and the American College of Obstetrics and Gynecology, each year we could save millions of dollars.

The only people who would stand to lose by terminating this "routine operation" would be the physicians who perform the procedure, and the hospitals that also charge for facilities and supplies. Assuming a busy obstetrical practice of 300 deliveries per year, half of these being males, an obstetrician, if he charged $200 per circumcision, would garner $30,000 per year. This is the price of a luxurious new car. If enterprising physicians could convince the American public of the need for female circumcision—after all, the female does possess a prepuce that accumulates smegma beneath it—they could realize an additional $30,000. For $60,000, one could purchase yearly the finest foreign car.

A recent study of Medicaid funding for circumcisions in the U.S. is instructive. Of the 34 states for which the annual Medicaid circumcision percentage rate could be determined, the circumcision rate in states that paid doctors less than $50 was 20.25%. In states that paid doctors more than $60, the circumcision rate nearly doubled to 38.04%. Is further proof needed to show that money drives circumcision?

It is interesting to note that when England switched to socialized medicine (1948) 53 years ago, circumcision was placed in the category of cosmetic surgery, and the physician was no longer reimbursed. The circumcision rate, which was high before socialization when physicians were monetarily compensated by insurance carriers, fell to below 0.5% when doctors were no longer paid for the operation.

- *Neonatal circumcision is the most frequently performed routine operation in the United States.*

- *Country-wide then, doctors are collecting as much as $240 million yearly to perform 1.2 million needless operations upon 1.2 million normal penises.*

- *In England, under socialized medicine when physicians were no longer compensated monetarily, the circumcision rate fell to below 1/2 of 1%.*

- *"The cost of circumcision varies geographically in the U.S. In L.A., obstetricians who perform the operation charge between $250 and $300. In Baltimore, physicians say the going rate is $150."*

  Parade Magazine,
  April 30, 1989

Victims' Voices . . .

"I was circumcised at birth, just because that was the way it was done in 1962. I'm a 26-year-old professional. I have often wondered what sex would be like if I had not been circumcised. It seems to me that it would be better if I had not had the operation. For example, if you worked all day with a glove on one hand and the other bare, you would have more feeling with the gloved hand, right? At any rate, I think it is done today for only two reasons—religion and doctors who want to make a fast buck off some poor uninformed parents. Hopefully, this will become a thing of the past."

S.C., New Mexico

30. Circumcision Does Not Prevent Premature Ejaculation

- *Premature ejaculation continues to be a common sexual complaint of American men, most of whom are circumcised.*

- *Proper attitude and communication remain the most important elements in sexual adjustment.*

Theoretically and actually, because the exposed circumcised glans penis has been toughened by years of abrasive contact with clothing, it should be, and is, less sensitive than the normal glans penis sheltered by the foreskin. On this basis alone, the circumcised male during intercourse should be slower in his buildup to orgasm. But several factors operate to modify this situation.

1. The physical act of intercourse sets into motion repetitive cyclic units of penile stimulation which prime the peri-urethral musculature culminating in orgasm. This factor certainly has some influence upon the time span of the sexual act.

2. But probably more important are the psychic factors, *attitudes and communications*, which emanates from that largest of sex organs, the *brain*. The manner in which we perceive our lover and ourself, our sense of fairness, sharing, generosity, love, trust, self-worth and respect, and past experiences—all these influence our act of love.

Premature ejaculation is a difficult problem to unravel. Its solution does not depend upon the presence or absence of a foreskin. It is probably equally common in circumcised and intact males. Psychic elements are probably more relevant to its occurrence and in its cure. Premature ejaculation continues to be a common sexual complaint of American men, most of whom are circumcised.

31. Penile and Cervical Cancer Are Not Valid Reasons for Infant Circumcision

Once I reached medical school, my thinking on circumcision was influenced by more universal, scientific reasoning. Now I was in a stronger position to more carefully evaluate facts pertaining to health. I discovered what every physician knows: medicine is not an exact science. There was frequently room for debate, skepticism, and bias. There are so many things relating to the human that we do not know. In medical school, matters pertaining to sex occupied but a minuscule part of our time. We did not have any formal course relating to human sexuality. But no one believed that masturbation contributed to mental instability, and circumcisions were not done to forestall insanity. We knew that one could masturbate without fear of losing one's eyesight or growing hair upon one's palms. (There were, however, a number of us who wore glasses.)

A new reason was given to routinely circumcise all male infants: the fear of getting cancer of the penis or cancer of the cervix. In the 1930's and 1940's, numerous medical articles appeared attesting to the fact that cancer of the penis practically never occurred in males circumcised shortly after birth. Jewish males did not get cancer of the penis. It was also documented that orthodox Jewish women rarely got cancer of the cervix. Smegma, the substance that might appear under the foreskin, was thought to contain a carcinogen. Circumcision was viewed as innocuous, with minimal complications, and no adverse aftereffects. Cancer obviously can be eventually fatal. So let us circumcise every newborn male and prevent cancer of the penis and cancer of the cervix. The idea made sense!

Home deliveries were no longer in vogue. The circumcision rate of hospital-delivered males hit close to 100% in a short period of time. Everyone was happy. Everyone's penis acquired the new "bald look" and doctors were making a few extra dollars on each male child delivered.

But things were not quite idyllic in the circumcision world. There were problems with circumcision. An occasional infant would bleed to death. There were infections. Many penises were deformed. There were serious complications.

And it turned out, cancer of the penis is a rare disease in the United States, and occurs usually in the lower socio-economic bracket in males totally ignoring sensible washing of the genitals.

Dr. James Snyder, past President of the Virginia Urological Society, notes that the low incidence of penile cancer in the United States is not due to circumcision because "... the population of American men born before 1940, now in the group at risk for this cancer, is a group of predominantly uncircumcised men." Research indicates that good hygiene prevents penile cancer and, according to Dr. Sydney Gellis, "It is an uncontestable fact...there are more deaths from circumcision each year than from cancer of the penis."

Soap and water confer the same protection against cancer of the penis as circumcision. The incidence of cancer of the penis in Europe, where circumcision is hardly done at all, is no higher than in the United States where it is done almost routinely.

Orthodox Jewish women may have a specific, genetic immunity to cancer of the cervix. Non-Jewish women have a relatively high incidence of cancer of the cervix even though most of their husbands are circumcised. And we now know that smegma is not carcinogenic.

So we were back to square one! I could never accept this idea of circumcising every male child to forestall cancer of the penis and/or cervix. Personally I hadn't seen smegma since the time I was a child, and I knew that this same situation applied to every other sensible, civilized man. I feel it an insult to presume that a child who would grow up to trim his fingernails, blow his nose, brush his teeth, and clean his

- *Soap and water confer the same protection against cancer of the penis as does circumcision.*

- *The incidence of cancer of the penis in Europe, where circumcision is hardly done at all, is no higher than in the United States where it is done almost routinely.*

- *Smegma, like sebum, is not carcinogenic.*

- *In the United States it requires the amputation of approximately 99,999 infant foreskins in order to save one old man who practices poor genital hygiene from ever developing cancer of the penis.*

- *Cancer of the cervix is no greater in Europe, where neonatal circumcision is **not** peformed.*

- *"Fatalities caused by circumcision accidents may approximate the mortality rate from penile cancer.... Perpetuating the mistaken belief that circumcision prevents cancer is inappropriate."*
  Letter from American Cancer Society (ACS) to AAP

31. *(continued)*
Penile and Cervical Cancer Are Not Valid Reasons for Infant Circumcision

anus, would be too stupid to learn how to retract the foreskin and to wash the glans penis—a procedure no more difficult nor demanding in time than washing a finger. This entire categorizing of males as so lacking in common sense relative to penile hygiene is preposterous and insulting. If one can believe the chauvinistic propaganda foisted upon us by the news media, there have even been males who have learned to tie their shoelaces and fly to the moon. The rate of cancer of the penis in the United States in our circumcised male population is about 1 to 2 cases/100,000 males. The rates in nearly all parts of Europe are similar. In England, Scandinavia, Germany, and Switzerland—and in South America and Japan—where circumcision is the exception, the incidence of cancer of the cervix is about the same, or less, than in the United States, where circumcision is routine.

Studies have revealed no difference in the incidence of cancer of the cervix among non-Jewish American women when comparing those married to circumcised men and those married to uncircumcised men.

Cancer of the cervix is a common and serious disease that may well be viral in origin. There may be a long latency period, possibly years, from the onset of an asymptomatic infection until its clinical manifestation years later. It probably occurs most commonly in: those initiating intercourse at an early age, those having multiple sex partners, those manifesting genital herpes, and those manifesting genital warts. Not enough time has elapsed to ascertain what impact HIV infections—AIDS—have upon the cause of cancer of the cervix.

32. The Intact Penis Is Not More Prone to Urinary Tract Infections

Recently, several medical studies have concluded that a circumcised child is less apt to get a urinary tract infection (UTI) than is a child with a normal, intact penis. These pro-circumcisionist allegations are diametrically contrary to sound, logical medical thinking. One is now to believe that amputating the foreskin and exposing the delicate glans penis, the urethra, and meatus to feces, urine-soaked diapers, and abrasive clothing is more healthful, and is less apt to cause infections of the urinary tract and the surrounding structures than is a normal intact glans penis and urethra shielded forever by the protective foreskin. This supposition is ludicrous and ridiculous.

Now more recently, the American Academy of Pediatrics reported that studies reflecting an increase in urinary tract infections among intact boys are "retrospective," may have "methodologic flaws," and "may have been influenced by selection bias." The more recent research of statistician and pediatrician, Dr. Martin Altschul, refutes the earlier UTI studies. New York pediatrician, Dr. Leonard J. Marino, agrees with Altschul: "Since one-fourth of my male infant patients are not circumcised, and if the frequency of UTI in the uncircumcised is as high as it is said to be, I should be seeing many UTIs in male infants. If I'm missing the diagnosis, they somehow are getting better without treatment. My experience reinforces the practice of discouraging routine circumcision, a cause of more morbidity than benefit."[11]

It is estimated that meatal ulceration (ulceration of the opening of the urethra) occurs in 20% to 50% of all circumcised infants, a complication that does not occur in the normal penis.

Meatal stenosis (stricture or narrowing) is an advanced degree of meatal ulceration and may occur in about one-third of all circumcised babies. With persistent or excessive ulceration, the tissue contracts and narrows the opening of the urethra, causing it to lose its normal slit-like, dumbbell-shaped contour, becoming round and sometimes pin-point. Varying degrees of urinary obstruction are possible. If the narrowing becomes too severe, a surgical meatotomy (enlarging of the end of the urethra with a scissors or a knife) may be necessary. This condition once again is iatrogenic (i.e. physician produced) and is not found in the normal penis protected by the foreskin. The stenosis may not be apparent for several years. Ironically, often the obstetrician, the individual who performed the circumcision and is responsible for this condition, does not have the benefit of patient follow-up, and is blithely ignorant of its existence.

Here is a partial list of additional infections that can result from neonatal circumcision:

  Tetanus (especially in Third World countries)
  Tuberculosis
  Meningitis
  Brain abscess
  Septicemia—generalized "blood poisoning"
  Osteomyelitis (infection of bones)
  Diphtheria

The contention that one will have fewer infections in an operated site, especially an area close to the anus, than in an intact normal skin surface defies logic.

- *Following circumcision, how does one prevent the glans penis from contacting feces, urine-soaked diapers, and abrasive clothing?*

- *"Since one-fourth of my male infant patients are not circumcised, and if the frequency of UTI in the uncircumcised is as high as it is said to be, I should be seeing many UTIs in male infants. If I'm missing the diagnosis, they somehow are getting better without treatment. My experience reinforces the practice of discouraging routine circumcision, a cause of more morbidity than benefit."*

  Leonard J. Marino, M.D.

- *Not only urinary tract infections, but* all *of the alleged reasons for doing a circumcision do not add up to justify doing it.*

  (See excerpts from AAP report after title page.)

33. The Intact Penis Is Not More Likely to Spread Sexually Transmitted Diseases, Including AIDS

- *An individual who depends upon a circumcised penis to protect himself against sexually transmitted diseases (STD) is indeed naive and foolhardy.*

- *People must be motivated towards responsible sexual activity and the avoidance of high risk sexual behavior. Anonymous sex and promiscuity must be abandoned.*

- *The fact is that the U.S. has one of the world's highest AIDS rate as well as the most circumcised sexually active males.*

- *"Our studies have not found circumcision to be either protective or a risk factor for AIDS or HIV infection in adults or in children."*
  Walter R. Dowdle, Ph.D.,
  Deputy Director (AIDS),
  Centers for Disease Control

An individual who depends upon a circumcised penis to protect himself against sexually transmitted diseases (STD) is indeed naive and foolhardy. Abstinence, of course, will guarantee a 100% method of protection. Short of abstinence, one must take one's chances. And the choice better be carefully made.

A generation ago, the traditional STD's numbered but five: syphilis, gonorrhea, chancroid, granuloma inguinale, and lymphopathia venereum. Now over two dozen STD's are recognized: 12 have bacterial origin; 8 are viral, 3 are protozoan, 1 is fungal, and 2 are ectoparasitic in origin. In the wake of the international AIDS epidemic, much of the emphasis on these other STD's has been weakened, if not lost. But STD's, aside from HIV (or AIDS) are still a frightening part of life. AIDS surpasses both cancer and rising medical care costs as the most serious health care problem facing Americans today. Even the near panic about genital herpes infections, so prominent a few years ago, has been relegated to minuscule importance.

But gonorrhea remains the most frequently reported infectious disease in the United States. Chlamydia is considered even more prevalent, and syphilis is resurgent.

Let us not forget that the antibiotics only have been available for about 40 plus years, and that without effective antibiotics, syphilis is one of the most easily contagious diseases known to man. Worldwide, the incidence of chancroid exceeds that of syphilis, and in Africa, the open sores of chancroid contribute to the rapid spread of HIV infections.

Antibiotics have fairly effectively controlled the STD's caused by bacteria, but according to the U.S. Centers for Disease Control (CDC) STD control for the balance of this century must focus on the primary prevention of all STD's, especially the persistent viral infections—including AIDS for which no therapies or vaccines currently exist. More emphasis must be placed on the concept of primary prevention, which we historically have tended to ignore. People must be motivated towards responsible sexual activity and the avoidance of high risk sexual behavior. Anonymous sex and promiscuity must be abandoned. A stable monogamous relationship must be adopted. Barrier contraceptions in conjunction with spermicides should be used. While domestically produced and FDA approved latex condoms may be the safest, bear in mind that 12% of American and 21% of foreign-made condoms failed the FDA leakage tests.

The myth that circumcision reduced the risk of STDs resulted from poorly designed studies published in the middle of the twentieth century. Newer studies have failed to document any consistent connection between the foreskin and STDs. Several of these studies have found that circumcised men are at greater risk for gonorrhea, chlamydial infections, and genital warts.

The AIDS epidemic is a frightening international tragedy. In a plague of this nature, sadly, there are those who play on public fears, prejudices, and ignorance.[12]

In the midst of this tragedy, urologist Aaron J. Fink, M.D., wrote to the New England Journal of Medicine to speculate that "the presence of a foreskin predisposes both heterosexual and homosexual men to the acquisition of AIDS."

To a reporter subsequently, Fink admitted, "This is nothing I can prove." (*United Press International*)

Based on this speculation by an ardent circumciser, several studies, mostly out of Africa, have looked for any connection between circumcision status and HIV infection. The results have been inconsistent. More often than

33. (continued) The Intact Penis Is Not More Likely to Spread Sexually Transmitted Diseases, Including AIDS

not, the study results reflect the circumcision status of the investigators. In many cases, study results can be attributed to other factors such as socioeconomic status, religion, tribal affiliation, and sexual practices. Based on the study designs employed to date, clearly identifying the role of circumcision in HIV infection is nearly impossible.

Circumcision enthusiasts have played up studies supporting their bias while ignoring studies refuting their position. Much of their promotion has taken place in the North American press in an effort to promote circumcision here, although they admit that the African HIV epidemic has little in common with the North American epidemic. These enthusiasts base nearly all of their claims of circumcision's protective effect on untested, unproven speculations. They also conveniently ignore the horrific complications reported commonly on the African continent. It is not known how many more African boys would die from circumcision if the practice increased there.

What these enthusiasts fail to realize is that the circumcision experiment has failed in the United States. Although the United States has the highest circumcision rate among developed nations, it also has the highest rates of HIV infection and other STDs. In comparison to western Europe, the rate of HIV infection acquired through heterosexual contact is 2 to 3 times higher. For example, the prevalence of heterosexually-acquired HIV is 39.8 per 100,000 in the United States, compared to 3.5 in Germany, 2.1 in Japan, 2.2 in Finland, 9.8 in Denmark, 11.9 in the Netherlands, 6.0 in Norway, and 7.3 in Sweden.† If circumcision was protective, one would expect the rate of HIV to be lower than in these similarly situated countries.

There is an epidemic of sexually transmitted diseases, including AIDS, in the United States where the majority of sexually active men are circumcised. It is not the foreskin that causes these diseases, and circumcision will not prevent them. "It is relatively more important to alter exposure to infectious agents than male susceptibility to them," wrote D.W. Cameron, M.D., FRCP. Cameron's AIDS research was erroneously and alarmingly reported by newspapers across the country with headlines which read, "Circumcision decreases risk of AIDS." Obviously, it is contact with specific organisms that causes specific diseases, and it is education about safe sex, not amputation of healthy body parts of newborns, that is sane preventive medicine for sexually transmitted diseases.

The spread of STDs including HIV is determined primarily by behavioral factors. When it comes to the transmission of infection, the amount of genital tissue is not nearly as important as to where that tissue is placed. As Paul Fleiss MD rhetorically proposed, "How much more of the penis must be amputated before transmission of HIV is made impossible?"* Most AIDS experts believe that in the absence of a vaccine the only viable means of controlling the HIV epidemic is to adequately address the behavioral elements fueling it. Even if one were to believe everything the circumcision enthusiasts assert, other interventions, such as aggressive treatment of STDs, have been demonstrated to be more effective, less costly, and have lower risk than the procedure the circumcision enthusiasts are proposing. From what is currently known, focusing any further attention on circumcision would be a waste of limited resources.

- *"It is not the foreskin that causes these diseases, and circumcision will not prevent them."*

    D.W. Cameron, M.D.

†Joint United Nations Programme on HIV/AIDS, World Health Organization. Global HIV/AIDS and STD Surveillance Project: Report on the global HIV/AIDS epidemic - June 1998.
*Fleiss PM. African apples, U.S. oranges. Pediatr News 1994; 28(11):19.

34. No, He Probably Won't Have to Have it Done Later Anyway

- *In Scandinavia, only two-tenths of one percent of older boys and men have to be circumcised for medical reasons.*

- *The U.S. military does not require or promote circumcision.*

- *Following adult circumcision, it takes several weeks until the glans "toughens," and contact with clothing is reasonably comfortable.*

- *"The rate of neonatal circumcision in Finland is zero, and the rate among older men is about 6 in 100,000."*

  Loraine Stern, M.D.

"It may have to be done later" is probably the most inane reason for infant circumcision. The issue of irresponsible prophylactic (preventative) surgery opens a Pandora's box of boundless nonsense. Extending this flawed logic to its obvious conclusion would strongly suggest removing all female infants' breasts. After all, 1 in 9 women will eventually develop breast cancer. Only 1 or 2 in 100,000 males develop penile cancer.

Let's take a look at Europe, where circumcision is not done on infants, and where physicians know the benefits of having a foreskin. Take Norway and Sweden, for example. There, only 1 in 500 older boys and men require circumcision for medical reasons. That's two-tenths of one percent.

There is another myth. It states that circumcision is mandatory for acceptance into the U.S. military. This is preposterous. For example, my brother, my cousins, and I were in the service, as were my three sons, one of whom was in the Air Force, one in the Army, and one in the Navy. And we all still have our foreskins.

Circumcision in the adult male is more involved than in the infant. The procedure is usually done in the operating room under general or spinal anesthesia, typically on an outpatient basis. A crushing clamp device cannot be used because the larger blood vessels cannot be securely occluded by mere crushing. They must be ligated (tied). But adult circumcision is relatively minor surgery. It's much less serious than an inguinal hernia or an appendectomy, for example. And although data is limited, adult circumcision probably has fewer complications than infant circumcision. It takes about 10 to 14 days for fairly good healing to occur. Often the now constantly exposed, hypersensitive glans must be protected (by cotton) for several weeks until the glans "toughens." As mentioned elsewhere in this book, circumcision represents a loss of about one-third of the normal skin covering the penis.

In the United States, approximately three circumcisions per year are performed for every 1,000 foreskin-intact adult males. These circumcisions of adults were for all reasons including personal preference, religious conversions, legitimate medical-surgical indications, etc. The United States rate is 50 times higher than in Finland where the circumcision rate in adult males is only 6/100,000. Worldwide, foreskin problems are treated medically, not surgically.

35. Intact Men Are More Likely to Use a Condom

A condom is used for two purposes: to prevent pregnancy, and to prevent the woman or man from contracting venereal disease. The objections to its use are that it is an impediment and break in the spontaneity and continuity in the act of making love, and it is thought to dull the pleasurable sensation resulting from covering the penis with a sheath. An objection that American males have to condom use is that they dull the sensations of intercourse. Much of this reaction may be due to the already dulled sensitivity of the glans penis as a result of circumcision and years of abrasion and dryness. Obviously, adding a layer of latex dulls the genital sensitivity even more.

But things are different for normal, intact males. Actually a lubricated condom does not detract one bit from the sensitivity of the normal intact penis. Imaginative couples might wish to incorporate its placement onto the penis with their love making.

Also because most American males lack a prepuce, the period of foreplay and dalliance may be abbreviated in the rush to the intra-vaginal method of penile stimulation. Both these factors conceivably could be of significance in increasing the rate of venereal disease, including AIDS, and unwanted teenage pregnancies. Incidentally, the United States has the highest rate of teenage pregnancies of any industrial nation. Shortening the period of foreplay would likewise be undesirable for most women.

- *Actually a lubricated condom does not detract one bit from the sensitivity of the normal intact penis.*

- *"Only one in three sexually active American girls between ages 15 and 19 uses contraceptives."*

  John Hopkins Research Group

36. Major Medical Associations Say Circumcision Is Unnecessary

- *Two other factors contribute to the risk of circumcision and its documentation. First, as medical personnel well know, many circumcisions are done by residents, not always the most experienced in this surgery, which requires some skill. Second, most circumcisions are done by obstetricians "who almost never see the patient again" and, consequently, miss seeing the complications.*

- *"There is no absolute medical indication for circumcision in the neonatal (newborn) period."*

    American Academy of Pediatrics, 1975

An increasing groundswell of oppositional awareness finally has prompted a number of national health groups to critically evaluate neonatal circumcision. In the 1970's, The American Academy of Pediatrics undertook such an evaluation. In 1971, and again in 1975, this group officially published its position.

"There is no absolute medical indication for routine circumcision of the newborn. The physician should provide parents with information pertaining to the long-term medical effects of circumcision and noncircumcision, so that they make a thoughtful decision. It is recommended that this discussion take place before the birth of the infant, so the parental consent to the surgical procedure, if given, will be truly informed.

"A program of education leading to continuing good personal hygiene would offer all the advantages of routine circumcision without the attendant surgical risk. Therefore, circumcision of the male neonate cannot be considered an essential component of adequate total health care." (American Academy of Pediatrics)

After reviewing recent studies which they admit are retrospective, may have methodologic flaws, and often contain conflicting evidence, the American Academy of Pediatrics in 1989 changed its 1975 statement to say "Newborn circumcision has potential medical benefits and advantages as well as disadvantages and risks." They did not say the potential benefits outweigh the known risks.[13]

Rarely-quoted excerpts from their 1989 report include:

- "Meatitis is more common in circumcised boys . . ."
- "Evidence regarding the relationship of circumcision to sexually transmitted diseases is conflicting."
- ". . . one study shows . . . a higher incidence of nonspecific urethritis in circumcised men."
- "Infants undergoing circumcision without anesthesia demonstrate physiologic responses suggesting they are experiencing pain."
- "The exact incidence of post-operative complications is not known . . ."
- "Local anesthesia adds an element of risk . . ."
- ". . . parents should be fully informed of the possible benefits and potential risks . . ."

Pediatricians treat the diseases of infants and children. Rarely do they perform circumcisions, but frequently they are confronted with problems that may arise from the operation. They are in a pivotal position to observe and recommend.

On the other hand, obstetricians—who along with general practitioners perform most circumcisions—seldom "follow-up" the male infants who they have circumcised. The obstetrical societies actually admonish their members not to treat male patients, and since most society members do not see the infant after the circumcision, they do not see the problems that may arise from its performance.

But obstetricians as a group also have taken a definite stand on the circumcision issue. In 1972, the American College of Obstetrics and Gynecology officially stated that there was no legitimate medical reason to circumcise every newborn male. Obstetricians in foregoing the procedure lose about $100 to $250 in their overall delivery fee. But their altruism transcends this monetary loss.

"The American College of Obstetricians and Gynecologists supports the conclusions of the AAP ad hoc Task Force on Circumcision (1975) that `there is no absolute medical indication for routine circumcision of the newborn.'

"The obstetrician is in a position of counseling parents in the prenatal and early neonatal period regarding circumcision. Facts should be presented to the parents so that they can make an informed decision. If the parents desire the procedure to be done, it is best performed during the neonatal period, after the first 12 to 24 hours. If parents decide against circumcision, then an educational effort by the baby's physician should be directed toward the parents concerning the normal anatomy, physiology, and care of the prepuce in early childhood."

In one Chicago area study, 50% of OB-GYN physicians are unaware of this policy statement by their own professional society. Many physicians, too, are failing to pass medical society policy information on to their patients. Also, it would seem that pediatricians and obstetricians are not communicating with one another very effectively.

In 1984, the American Academy of Pediatrics published a brochure entitled, "Care of the Uncircumcised Penis." In it some functions of the foreskin are detailed:

> "The function of the foreskin: the glans at birth is delicate and easily irritated by urine and feces. The foreskin shields the glans; with circumcision, this protection is lost. In such cases, the glans and especially the urinary opening (meatus) may become irritated or infected, causing ulcers, meatitis (inflammation of the meatus), and meatal stenosis (a narrowing of the urinary opening). Such problems virtually never occur in uncircumcised penises. The foreskin protects the glans throughout life." (Official statement and policy of the American Academy of Pediatrics: "Care of the Uncircumcised Penis," 1984)

Other prestigious groups have followed the lead of the pediatricians and obstetricians. John Hopkins University Hospital in 1982, and the University of Texas, to name a few, have announced that neonatal circumcision would no longer be performed unless specifically requested by the parents.

Why has circumcision continued at such a high rate in light of these official statements? Most likely because of the following:

1. Misinformation
2. Lack of communication
3. Tradition
4. Stubbornness
5. Money

---

36. *(continued)* Major Medical Associations Say Circumcision Is Unnecessary

- *In 1984, the American Academy of Pediatrics published a brochure entitled, "Care of the Uncircumcised Penis." In it some functions of the foreskin are detailed.*

37. Some Insurance Companies Are No Longer Paying for Routine Infant Circumcision

Another relevant item has entered the circumcision lists, cost! Medicine is in the era of cost containment. Health care insurance providers are scrutinizing the validity of practically all surgical procedures, and they have concluded, just as the pediatric and obstetrical societies have, that routine neonatal circumcision does not make sense either medically or monetarily. Pennsylvania Blue Cross and Blue Shield have sent their subscribers the following notices: "Pennsylvania Blue Shield will no longer cover routine neonatal circumcision... The decision to exclude coverage is based on medical research findings that the procedure is not beneficial." (January 1, 1987)

Nationwide, other Blue Cross-Blue Shield groups, in addition to many other medical insurance carriers, have taken the same action. The subscriber must pay for the operation out of his/her own pocket. It will be interesting to see how this situation impacts upon the number of circumcisions that are or are not done in the United States in the future.

In Canada, the circumcisions paid for by Provincial Health Agencies has declined from forty-four percent (44%) in 1975 to only four percent (4%) in 1995. Ten provincial and territorial health jurisdictions reached the same conclusion independently: paying for circumcisions can no longer be justified.

38. Many Noted Physicians and Others Have Spoken Out Against Circumcision

"My own preference, if I had the good fortune to have another son, would be to leave his little penis alone."[14]

Benjamin Spock, M.D.,
Author, *Baby and Child Care*

"Circumcision is a very cruel, very painful practice with no benefit whatsoever."

Ashley Montagu, Ph.D.

"In addition to the obvious discomfort involved, there are now serious concerns this routine procedure may actually deprive adult men of a vital part of their sexual sensitivity."

Dean Edell, M.D.,
National Radio Host

"All of the Western world raises its children uncircumcised and it seems logical that, with the extent of health knowledge in those countries, such a practice must be safe."[15]

C. Everett Koop, M.D.,
former Surgeon General

"Widespread circumcision is a relic of a time when patients were not provided much of a voice in medical decision-making. That era may be rapidly coming to an end. In this case, the old dictum that `if it ain't broke, don't fix it' seems to make good sense. Submitting your son to the procedure to prevent urinary infections makes only a little more sense than buying insurance against being gored by a unicorn in Riverside."[16]

Eugene Robin, M.D.,
Stanford University Medical School

"Even if you found that there were absolutely no harmful psychological effects, it would still not justify doing an unnecessary procedure. You just should not be cruel to babies."

Paul Fleiss, M.D.,
University of Southern California
Medical School

"My feeling is that it is a traumatic experience and I am opposed to traumatizing the baby. I'm also opposed to inflicting an operation on an individual without his permission. My feelings became more concrete when I talked to Dr. Leboyer and saw his birth film. It seemed so incongruous to have a non-violent birth and then immediately do violence to the baby by circumcising him."

Howard Marchbanks, M.D.
Family Practitioner

"In response to circumcision, the baby cries a helpless, panicky, breathless, high-pitched cry! Another thing which sometimes happens with babies who are being circumcised is that they can lapse into a semi-coma. People don't distinguish between that high-pitched, panicky, breathless cry and a normal loud cry. And people don't make the distinction between sleep and semi-coma. Both of these states, helpless crying and semi-coma, are abnormal states in the newborn."

Dr. Justin Call, Infant Psychologist,
Professor-in-Chief of Child and
Adolescent Psychology,
University of California-Irvine

"The ... American doctors who still perform circumcision are violating the first rule of good medical care--primum non nocere—first, do no harm. Few ... really understand what they are doing when they amputate the foreskin, for they have never studied how the penis develops before birth. Since the penis is used for procreation only a few times in the entire life of the individual, sexual pleasure must also be one of its major functions, and the foreskin is an integral part of that sexual pleasure."

George Denniston, M.D.
University of Washington,
School of Medicine

"Thousands of men with AIDS fill the hospital beds of our major cities and are testimony to the failure of circumcision to offer any degree of immunity to AIDS infections. No one seriously advocates removing the breasts of female infants to prevent this more common malignancy of breast cancer. Circum-

38. *(continued)*
Many Noted Physicians and Others Have Spoken Out Against Circumcision

cision must be recognized as an equally serious mutilation of men with equally insubstantial justification for continuing the practice.

"The risks of newborn circumcision are an under-reported and ignored factor in this argument. Most often a poor surgical result is not recognized until years after the event. By the time a child reaches the age of maturity and discovers how he has been mistreated, the surgeon cannot be found, and parents may be beyond the age of interest in such matters. The child who simply has been cut too short will then become a sexually dysfunctional adult."

James Snyder, M.D., Past President, Virginia Urologic Society

"Whatever is done to stop the terrible practice of circumcision will be of tremendous importance. There is no rational, medical reason to support it. And, much worse, no one is aware of the deep implications and life-lasting effect. The torture is experienced in a state of total helplessness which makes it even more frightening and unbearable. It is high time that such a barbaric practice comes to an end."

Dr. Frederick Leboyer, Author, *Birth Without Violence*

"Cutting off this structure (the foreskin) is possibly the oldest human sexual ritual. It still persists—on the ground, now, either that cancer of the penis and cervix is rarer when it is done (washing probably works as well) or that it slows down orgasm (for which there is no evidence). We're against it, though for some it is already too late. 'To cut off the uppermost skin of the secret parts,' said Dr. Bulwer 'is directly against the honesty of nature, and an injurious insufferable trick put upon her.' The point is that if you have a foreskin, you conserve your options. It probably doesn't make very much difference, either to masturbation or to intercourse, but it makes some, and nobody wants to lose a sensitive structure. Normally one retracts it anyway for all these purposes, but if you haven't one there is a whole range of covered-glans nuances you can't recapture."

Alex Comfort, M.D., *The New Joy of Sex*

"It is important to know the structure of any organ before we ablate it (before we cut it off and destroy it). This would . . . make good sense."

John Taylor, M.D.

"The fact is that the 'foreskin' is not a separate anatomical structure, but rather a continuous part of the penile skin system. Infant circumcision actually removes about 25% to 60% of the skin of the entire penis, not some separate structure called the 'foreskin.'"

Francisco Garcia
Medical Student

"Although a commonly performed procedure, the true incidence of complications associated with this procedure is at best an estimate. These complications are often overlooked or under-reported. According to Gee and Ansell's excellent review, most complications were discovered only by carefully examining the nurses' notes."

Dr. John Gearhart
Urologic Complications Chapter 31

"The U.S. Armed Forces advocated circumcision because it gave an opportunity for young surgeons to practice . . . Circumcision was felt to promote discipline. I presume as a result of a young recruit's learning what the Army could do to him at the onset, he might be influenced to behave himself."

Dr. Mendelson

"It is an incontestable fact that there are more deaths each year from complications of circumcision than from cancer of the penis."

Dr. Sydney Gellis

"We in the United States are culturally acclimated to regard the foreskin as nonessential and even pathologic. We must not forget that the burden of proof is on the circumcision advocates. [To justify removing it,] they must show cause and effect."

Martin Altschul, M.D.
Pediatrician

"The primary function of the foreskin is . . . to allow vaginal inter-

38. (continued) Many Noted Physicians and Others Have Spoken Out Against Circumcision

"course to take place under optimal conditions without friction between the mucosal surfaces of the participants."
Dr. Michael Beauge

"A survey of physicians revealed that 60% of those polled did not know the purpose of the prepuce (foreskin)."
Martin Stein, M.D.

"When women want to enlarge a perfectly normal organ, the breast, they've gotten support, and even encouragement. But when men want to restore a perfectly normal and useful part of their bodies, that was removed from them against their will, [some doctors tell them] they have to undergo psychiatric exams . . . This is a sad incongruous truism."
Dr. Dean Edell,
Well-known Radio and TV Commentator

"My family's experience . . . is . . . my father telling our Jewish physician he is not to touch his son in any way. The physician seemed to discount what my father said and I vividly remember my father grabbing they physician by the shirt collar, invading his space, glaring him eye to eye, and obtaining the physician's agreement that he would not 'touch' my brother. Nonetheless, still unknown to my family . . . our Jewish physician did a Synechia-lysis, and I remember my mother having explicit instructions on how to care for my brother. I remember how inflamed and painful it seemed to be to my brother . . . There is a compulsive inability to leave infants alone. The compulsive issue must be explored and addressed."
Eileen Wayne, M.D.

"Any . . . mother who is 'eccentric enough' to wish her child to retain his prepuce would be well advised to maintain permanent guard over it . . . ."
William Keith Morgan, M.D.

Were girls so treated, there would be widespread protests. In my opinion, the socially tolerated abuse of males is one of the primary causes of unconscious male rage and violence.
Aaron Kipnis, Ph.D.
Male Privilege or Privation?

"I feel that there's no solid medical evidence at this time to support routine circumcision. Some parents may choose circumcision for religious reasons. In other cases, I recommend leaving the foreskin the way Nature meant it to be."
Michael B. Rothenberg, M.D.
Co-author, with Dr. Benjamin Spock of Dr. Spock's Baby and Child Care, 6th Edition 1992

" . . . Physicians who assume responsibility for the health of male patients for operative or other care, will not be regarded as specialists in obstetrics-gynecology . . . "
American Board of Obstetrics and Gynecology Inc. 1976

"The best way to stop the complications of circumcision is to stop doing them."
Mitch Ryder, M.D.

"Only be denying the existence of excruciating pain, perinatal encoding of the brain with violence, interruption of maternal-infant bonding, betrayal of infant trust, the risks and effects of permanently altering normal genitalia, the right of human beings to sexually intact and functional bodies, and the right of individual religious freedoms can human beings continue this practice."
Marilyn Fayre Milos, RN and Donna Macris CNM, MSN

"Lying outside the province of modern surgery, however, the procedure frequently features illogical bases for patient selection, neglect of the requirement to obtain informed consent, an inappropriate operator, needlessly radical technique, disregard for pain, dubious objectives, and unknown cost-effectiveness."
David Grimes, M.D.
Professor, OB/GYN
University of CA, San Francisco

"I will prescribe regimen for the good of my patients according to my ability and my judgment, and never do harm to anyone."
Hippocrates

39. If You're Not Sure—Don't Do It!

There is one clearing house organization you can contact if you want to talk to someone or read more about circumcision:

> National Organization of Circumcision
> Information Resource Centers (NOCIRC)
> National Headquarters (call for nearest office)
> P.O. Box 2512
> San Anselmo, CA 94979
> (415) 488-9883
> (415) 488-9660 (Fax)

When you do decide against circumcision and for a whole, natural penis, it may be wise to use a letter like the sample shown below to notify your physician and hospital.

Date: _____
Maternal and Newborn Care Staff:
Hospital: _____
Address: _____
_____

Dear (Doctor or Hospital):

I/We, _____ are expectant parent(s) who plan to give birth to our child while under your care.

This communication is to notify you that, should our child be a boy, he is NOT to be circumcised under any circumstances. We oppose the practice of routine circumcision of newborn male infants.

To avoid any possible potential for inadvertent "accidental" slip up whereby our son could possibly be accidentally circumcised, we hereby request that the mother's chart be immediately marked upon admission, that the child's chart, if a boy, be immediately marked as well as his nursery crib be marked: **Circumcision Not Authorized**.

We further request that no attempt be made by any medical staff or attendant to stretch, retract, or otherwise forcibly attempt to retract or manipulate our baby's prepuce (foreskin).

Thank you for your attention to these concerns.

Sincerely yours,

Permission to copy and use this letter is hereby granted.

40. Say No to Circumcision!

For many millions of Americans, the message of this book has come too late to influence their genital status. But surely the prudent man and woman will act with wisdom and altruism in decisions affecting the future happiness of their children.

Hopefully, after reading this book, one will "now know" and therefore "see" the rational approach to this issue of routine newborn circumcision of our males.

I close with this thought from Socrates, "The object of our discussion is not that your words may gain victory over mine, or that mine may triumph over yours, but that together, we may discover the perfect truth."

- *"One sees what one knows."*
  Goethe

- *"The object of our discussion is not that your words may gain victory over mine, or that mine may triumph over yours, but that together, we may discover the perfect truth."*
  Socrates

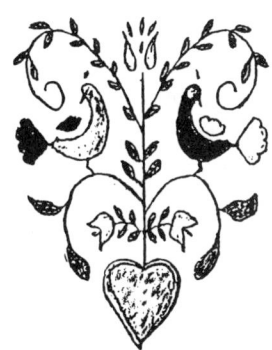

Glossary

Cavernous Bodies: Vascular (blood vessel) spaces in the erectile bodies of the clitoris and penis that trap blood during sexual congress causing these bodies to enlarge and to erect.

Circumcision: The amputation of all or part of the foreskin (prepuce) of the male or female. (See Infibulation.)

Coitus, Coital: Sexual intercourse.

Corona: The prominent elevated rim which is the base of the glans penis.

Clitoris: A small, elongated, erectile sensory structure at the forward part of the vulvar (vaginal) lips.

Dehiscence: The act of splitting or rupturing beyond its normal boundary.

Dilate: To stretch beyond its normal dimensions.

Distal: Farther from the center (of the body).

Dorsum, Dorsal: The back, or pertaining to the back of a structure, e.g. the top of one's own penis that one sees when looking down upon it. (The under surface of the penis is the ventral surface.)

Ejaculation: The act of expulsion of semen through the urethra.

Etiology: The study or theory of the causation of any disease.

Fistula: A tunnel-like defect in tissue possessing an entrance and an exit.

Flaccid: Weak; lax; soft, e.g. an unerect penis.

Foreskin: The prepuce. The loose retractable skin sheath at the end of the natural penis or clitoris.

Frenulum: The cord-like structure on the under (ventral) side of the glans penis that connects the glans to the foreskin (similar to the structure at the base of the human tongue).

Glans: The distal end, or terminal rounded end of the clitoris or penis.

Infibulation: The fastening together of the female's genital lips so as to create a mechanical barrier to intercourse. (This more radical genital mutilation is often performed.)

Intact: Untouched; uninjured, e.g. an uninjured, normal penis; an intact hymen or eardrum.

Keratin: The dry, sometimes horny material that forms on skin or mucosal surfaces in response to excessive friction and exposure, or to the deprivation of sebum or smegma.

Masturbate: Self-genital stimulation and pleasuring.

Meatotomy: The cutting of the urinary (urethral) meatus (opening) in order to enlarge it.

Meatus: A passage or opening; especially the orifice (opening) of the end of the male's urethra.

Mortality: The death rate.

Morbidity: The condition of being diseased or morbid. The sick rate.

Necrosis: The death of a segment of tissue.

Neonatal: Used interchangeably with newborn.

Neuro-vascular corpuscles: Minute sensory organs composed of nerve and vascular tissue, which, when stimulated, produce pleasure.

Orgasm: The climax of sexual excitement in intercourse.

Orifice: An opening through which something (e.g. urine, semen) may pass.

Perineum: The diamond-shaped area on the underside of the male and female torso through which pass the genitals and the anus.

Periurethral: The muscles surrounding the base of the male urethra, under voluntary and reflex control.

Phimosis: Inability to retract the foreskin after the age of puberty.

Prepuce, Preputial: Foreskin and/or pertaining to the foreskin.

Proximal: Nearer to the center of the body.

Sebum: The (somewhat greasy) secretion of the sebaceous glands.

Semen: The thick, whitish liquid produced by the testes, prostate, etc. ejaculated in intercourse.

Smegma: Desquamated epithelial cells and sebum; the harmless, protective, lubricating secretion (very similar to sebum) found under the foreskin of the penis and clitoris and about the labia minora.

Stenosis: Narrowing of a structure, e.g. the urethral (urinary) meatus.

STD: Sexually transmitted disease.

Stricture: The abnormal narrowing of a passageway either by scar contracture or a deposit of abnormal tissue.

Sulcus: A groove, trench, or furrow, e.g. the coronal sulcus of the penis (the groove that encircles the penis where the glans meets the penile shaft).

Transect: To cut across.

Trauma: Any wound or injury.

Turgid: Swollen and/or congested, e.g. an erect penis.

Urethra: The tube-like conduit (for urine and/or semen) that connects the bladder to the exterior of the body.

UTI: Urinary tract infections.

Vascular: Pertaining to blood vessels.

Ventral: The "belly" or front side of the body. Also the under surface of the penile shaft.

Vulva: The visible external parts of the female genitalia.

Physicians Guide to the Normal (Intact) Penis

The material in this appendix has been requested by numerous American physicians because there is so much misinformation on this subject in the medical literature.

Introduction

The foreskin of the human male's penis should not be removed at birth except in rare instances. In Finland, where the circumcision rate is zero at birth, the risk of needing the foreskin removed later is one in sixteen thousand, six hundred sixty seven (1/16,667), an extremely rare event![1] The prepuce is invariably normal and almost never requires removal.

The prepuce is an integral part of the human penis, as it is of all mammalian penises. This highly specialized region of mucous membrane and skin has several important functions. All of the reasons given to justify removal have turned out to be invalid. The risk of a myriad of complications far outweighs any alleged "benefits." And no one has the right to remove an important normal part of someone else's body.

Care and Development of the Intact Penis

Proper hygiene for the intact male is extremely simple. Here are the basic rules:

1. Leave the foreskin alone![2]

The major function of the foreskin during the early years is to protect the glans and urinary opening. If the infant can urinate, there is usually nothing to worry about.

2. Never permit anyone to retract the foreskin.

While it remains attached, the foreskin is the skin of the glans. It is there to *protect* the glans. Retraction can tear the attachment, producing pain, scarring and disfigurement. When left alone, separation occurs naturally.

If a young man is unable to retract his foreskin as a teenager, it is still, although less common, perfectly normal.

3. When the child can fully retract his own foreskin comfortably, he may begin to do so in the tub or shower.

A little clear water, running over the retracted prepuce and exposed glans, is all the hygiene that is necessary. Let us look at these rules in more detail:

Leave the Foreskin Alone

The intact male has a glans penis that is an internal organ. It is still fully covered with skin, and, at birth in 96% of male infants, the foreskin is incapable of full retraction without damaging the penis.

During intra-uterine life, the foreskin completely covers and is inseparable from the glans penis. Before an infant is born, the process of separation of the foreskin from the glans begins, but in almost all infants, it is not complete at birth. Many foreskins are still not fully retractable at puberty; a few continue to be non-retractable at the age of 17 years.

Never Permit Anyone to Retract the Foreskin

This warning is given to mothers and to anyone caring for a male infant. Numerous nurses and doctors, having failed to understand the normal penis, have been known to retract the foreskin forcibly.[3] When this is done, the beautiful mechanism that protects the glans is threatened, and the skin is literally torn off the rest of the organ. The infant or child screams and scarring of the glans and prepuce results. Mothers need to warn doctors, nurses and others *before* an intact child is examined not to retract. If forced retraction does occur, it may be treated with a topical steroid rather than circumcision.[4]

Forcible retraction of the prepuce by medical personnel has been cause for successful legal action.

Let the Child Retract His Own Foreskin

Let the child retract his own foreskin over time, and, as it naturally becomes quite loose, hygiene will consist simply of running water over the glans and foreskin.

Prepuce "Problems" and How to Care for Them

"Patience and time! Patience and time!"[5] A useful prescription for many penile problems.

Ammonia Dermatitis

If an infant develops a reddened foreskin, it may be an infection. Cutting through infected tissue to remove it is dangerous. Most commonly, a reddened foreskin is an ammoniacal dermatitis. Ammonia is produced by a specific bacterium in the infant's feces, B.ammoniagenes. The ammonia causes the reddening, which may extend over the diapered area, and may include vesicles and papules with some excoriation. The lesions are stopped by treating the diapers with an antiseptic (mercuric chloride), which inhibits the ammonia-producing bacterium.[6] Circumcision is contraindicated.

Allergy to Alkali in Soap

Another irritation of the foreskin may be stopped by discontinuing the use of soap. Simply wash the penis with warm water —nothing more—and, with patience and time, the redness disappears.[7] Circumcision is contraindicated.

Ballooning of the Foreskin

If, at any time during childhood, the opening remains small, while the urine stream is considerable, the foreskin may balloon, with urine under back-pressure. This is normal, so long as urination is not markedly prolonged. Circumcision is contraindicated.

Decreased Urinary Stream

If the urine comes out as a mist, and urination is prolonged, steps may be taken to remedy the situation. A local anesthetic may be applied to the foreskin. After one hour, the foreskin is pulled forward until the urinary meatus is visualized. Then 1% hydrocortisone cream is sparingly applied six times a day for four weeks, and once or twice a day for two weeks after that. Accompany this cream with gentle retraction, preferably by the boy himself. Circumcision is contraindicated.

Forced Retraction of Tight Foreskin (Paraphimosis)

Take care not to pull the still tight foreskin back beyond the base of the glans. If this is done, it acts like a tourniquet. Blood can get into the glans, but it cannot easily get out. If this condition occurs, and is discovered promptly, the situation can easily be treated with gentle, prolonged hand pressure using a well-lubricated glove, squeezing the glans gently until the blood is forced out of it, and the foreskin can be pulled over it.

Pinhole Opening in Foreskin

If one were to look gently for the opening in the tip of the infant foreskin, it is often found to be a "pinhole" in size. Yet, while the adult is still looking, and gently manipulating the penis, it is not uncommon for the infant to release a stream of urine. The size of the outlet becomes considerably larger than the visualized pinhole. This extraordinary disparity in the size of the opening, depending on whether pressure is applied from the outside or the inside, vividly documents the primary function of the foreskin at this time in the infant's life—that of *protection*, while still permitting function. The infant can urinate normally, but the pinhole opening is an effective part of the foreskin barrier.

Smegma

The white material that collects under the prepuce is called smegma. Smegma is formed as the result of a natural process. Skin is always renewing itself by sloughing off dead cells. Smegma is little more than those dead cells: like the material that one obtains by scratching the forearm with a fingernail, or that collects between the toes. During childhood, smegma is a product of the process whereby the preputial space is formed.

In the child, smegma should be left alone. Much confusion arises while trying to determine when to retract the foreskin for cleansing.[8] At such time as the child is able to retract his own foreskin comfortably, he can let water run over the penis. That is the full extent of hygiene required for a child's, and for an adult's, penis.

Smegma tends to increase at puberty. This is perfectly normal.

The Functions of the Foreskin

The foreskin has several useful functions: it serves to protect the infant glans and urethra from feces and other sources of infection. In the infant, and in the adult as well, the protecting foreskin prevents the thin mucous membrane surface of the glans from thickening. Without protection, the glans adds numerous layers of cells with a consequent loss of sensitivity. When this thickening occurs around the urethral meatus, it produces meatal stenosis, or narrowing, a common complication of circumcision, often requiring further surgical intervention to open it.[9] In addition, meatal ulceration with scarring is also common.

The foreskin eventually separates from the surface of the glans. During erection, the penile shaft elongates, becoming about 50% longer and the separated foreskin covers this lengthened shaft. It develops to accommodate the penis, which is capable of a marked increase in diameter and length. Removing the foreskin leads to tightness, discomfort, and even penile curvature.

In addition to its function in normal erection, the foreskin makes masturbation, now recognized as a completely normal activity, easier and much more pleasurable.

The foreskin makes it easier for the male to enter the female. During entry, the foreskin slides back, as nature intended. This function may be compared with the rolling on of a condom. No one tries to pull an unrolled condom on. The friction is too great.

The foreskin has complex nerve endings, described by Taylor, which give a degree of sexual pleasure not experienced without it.[10] Some twenty small concentric, circumferential ridges, collectively called the frenar band, carry specialized nerve endings back and forth across the corona of the glans, producing pleasure. One man, who had a circumcision *after* he had become sexually active, said: "Stimuli that had previously aroused ecstasy now have relatively little effect."

An intact foreskin, properly cared for, is a pleasure that all humans have a right to enjoy.

Intact Children Require Parental Protection: "Leave my son alone!"

American parents with intact sons must realize that they may have difficulty while their sons are growing up in protecting them from mutilation. Sometimes doctors have difficulty protecting their own sons. In America today, parents of intact sons must remain alert.

The foreskin can cover the glans completely without ever being retractable. Though rare, this is perfectly normal. Many men prefer this to circumcision. Of course, it is more usual for the tip of the foreskin to gradually enlarge, and for the remaining attachment points between the foreskin and the glans to dissolve. By puberty, many boys have a fully retractable foreskin, which can easily be pulled back so the glans is fully exposed. There is no constriction, because the foreskin is now a wide channel.

At puberty, many boys cannot fully retract their foreskin. This is no cause for alarm. It is perfectly normal. By age 17, most boys can retract, but even then, non-retractability is not sufficient reason to circumcise.

Excuses that Doctors Use to Circumcise

Around 1860, doctors suggested that circumcision would prevent masturbation. As soon as that absurd idea was dismissed, they found another excuse. And so it continues . . .

Hygiene

Most Americans have rarely seen an intact penis. If they have, it has been the penis of an infant whose foreskin normally extends well beyond the tip of the glans and is gathered tightly around it. They have difficulty imagining that this foreskin, if left alone, will enlarge and expand with normal growth to become a loose-fitting arrangement during childhood. They scarcely realize that any intact male can gently pull his foreskin back and look as if he were circumcised. At that point, cleansing is identical for the circumcised and the intact.

Cancer of the Penis

Another excuse has been that circumcision prevents cancer of the penis. This type of cancer occurs in one in *one hundred thousand* (1/100,000) men. Who could reasonably suggest that circumcision be done on all male infants to prevent this extremely rare cancer of the adult penis? For comparison, the risk of breast cancer is now about one in nine (1/9), yet no one suggests we remove all female breasts at puberty to prevent this formidable disease.

Gairdner's study was instrumental in stopping circumcision in Great Britain during the 1950s. His data showed there would be 15 infant deaths from circumcision each year per one hundred thousand circumcisions.[11] Who wants to risk killing 15 infants to possibly prevent one cancer of the penis in one older man?

Because of its rarity, is it not unethical to mention cancer of the penis as a "reason" for circumcising?

Urinary Tract Infection

Recently, the excuse for circumcising has been the alleged prevention of urinary tract infections. Thomas Wiswell, M.D., has claimed that 1% of intact boys get urinary tract infections. Even if we accept Wiswell's facts, which wiser doctors disagree with, it is only 1% of intact infants who get urinary tract infections. No doctor should justify harming 100 infants to possibly protect one of them from an infection that is normally treated with antibiotics. All European doctors treat these infections without resorting to circumcision. In view of the extremely low incidence of urinary tract infection in the intact newborn, is it not unethical to mention UTI's as a "reason" for circumcising?

Prevention of Sexually-Transmitted Diseases (STDs)

In America, it is not customary for parents to decide how their children will conduct themselves sexually. Parents can neither predict, nor control, their children's sexual behavior. Therefore, even if foreskin removal did prevent STDs, the intact young person might prefer to choose avoiding exposure.

The idea that circumcision does prevent STDs is ludicrous. Simply look at the incidence of STDs in a country (USA) that has a majority of its males circumcised! Rather, we should ask, can we prove that circumcision does not increase the risk of STD?

Cancer of the Cervix

An excellent paper by Terris demonstrates that there is no increased risk of cancer of the cervix in the partners of intact men.[12] A physician in another study determined that the circumcision status of the partner (because the woman often did not know). No association between cancer of the cervix and circumcision status was found.[13] In Europe, where circumcision is not performed, cancer of the cervix is no higher than in the U.S. Cancer of the cervix is simply another excuse for circumcision that has never been proven.

Do circumcision now, because it might otherwise have to be performed later. In Finland, the rate of post-neonatal circumcision is one in sixteen thousand six hundred and sixty-seven men (1/16,667).[14] This figure demonstrates how incredibly normal the foreskin is, and provides some indication of the vast numbers of unnecessary, indeed, contraindicated circumcisions still being done in the United States.

Phimosis

Phimosis is a normal condition of the human prepuce in young males. The word comes directly from the Greek and means "muzzling." Its English definition is "A tightness or constriction of the orifice of the prepuce, arising either congenitally or from inflammation, congestion, etc, and making it impossible to bare the glans." This, of course, is precisely what the prepuce does during the early years of life. The ending, "-osis," according to Webster's International Dictionary, means a suffix signifying "condition, state, process." A condition of muzzling. Perfectly normal.

Dr Peter Lord, Secretary of the Royal College of Surgeons, says, ". . . Phimosis does not occur with a healthy foreskin. A high proportion of small boys are not able to retract their foreskin until six, and sometimes later. ..no harm at all in leaving it unretracted to that age, unless of course there is recurrent infection [see Balanitis]. Usually by the age of five or six the little fellow is sufficiently interested in his anatomy to have done some exploring and to have found that he can retract. If, however, he falls into the hands of the School Doctor, or the District Nurse, he may be referred to the Surgeon with a view to circumcision for phimosis.[15]

Paraphimosis

Para comes from the Greek and means "associated in a subsidiary capacity." Paraphimosis refers to the situation where a constricted prepuce is retracted, baring the glans. The constricted prepuce acts like a tourniquet on the penile shaft. With constriction, swelling of the glans occurs and gangrene could ultimately result, unless it is promptly reduced, as described in the section titled, "Forced retraction of tight foreskin."

Balanitis

Literally, "inflammation of the acorn" or glans penis, diagnosis of balanitis requires redness, swelling and pus. Beware of the diagnosis of balanitis, which is not really balanitis, but simply irritation (redness) and normal smegma. Balanitis does not cause phimosis, and no single pathogen is involved. Usually a boy suffers only one episode.[16] Balanitis may be treated by bathing in hot water, local washing, or like other infections—with antibiotics. In the case of candidal balanitis, acidophilus culture is indicated and fungicides may be used.[17] Balanitis has often been used as an excuse to circumcise.

Balanoposthitis

Inflammation of the glans and prepuce. Treatment consists of diagnosis of the offending organism(s), and appropriate antibiotic therapy, not removal of the organ.

Preputial Stenosis (Balanitis xerotica obliterans)

This rare disease of unknown etiology, which rarely occurs before age 5, exists only when there is cicatrization of the preputial orifice with histologic changes of balanitis xerotica obliterans (BXO). It is characterized by a thick white fibrous ring around the prepuce, and by pale gray, parchment-like skin. There is thinning of the epidermis, and replacement of the dermis with dense collagenous tissue infiltrated with chronic inflammatory cells. The epidermis separates easily from the dermis.[18] This condition can be progressive. Since, in the adult, the likelihood of the progression of the disease to involve the anterior urethra may be increased by circumcision, since spontaneous regression may occur, and since the changes of BXO have been reversed by the local application of corticosteroids,[19] it would be well to consider conservative treatment before resorting to circumcision.[20,21]

Preputial Adhesions

Under normal conditions, preputial adhesions do not exist. The prepuce is not adherent to the glans; the prepuce is the skin of the glans, initially attached just as tightly as the skin on one's finger. At birth, a space has begun to form between the prepuce and the glans, the preputial space, and the process of creating this space is not yet complete.

At approximately 17 weeks gestation, cells in the area of separation between the future foreskin and the glans initiate the process of creating the preputial space. They begin to form microscopic balls comprising multiple layers of cells. As these whorls of cells enlarge, cells at the center are cut off from nutrients; they die and create a space. These minute spaces coalesce, eventually becoming the preputial space. Some boys will not have a fully retractable foreskin until after puberty.

The preputial space will inevitably become complete without outside interference. When a doctor begins a circumcision, he will usually take a probe, and run it around in this partially formed space, disrupting the attachments between the two organs, the prepuce and the glans. Now adhesions can truly form because raw surfaces remain on both organs after this disruption.

Redundant Foreskin

Sometimes in the infant, the foreskin may seem excessive beyond the tip of the glans. This is perfectly normal because the entire organ is going to grow and change. In the boy, this so-called extra skin will begin to serve one of its most important functions. It slides down to cover the enlarging shaft of the penis during an erection.

Hypospadias

Hypospadias refers to the urethral opening not exiting at the tip of the glans, as it usually does, but below the tip, somewhere along the underside of the penis. This condition arises through a failure of normal development. Circumcision is contraindicated in such cases because urologic surgeons currently use the foreskin to make the repair.

Since it is virtually impossible to make the diagnosis until a circumcision is under way, or until time permits normal unforced retraction of the foreskin, circumcision should never be contemplated until the diagnosis can be made without risk of harming the child (through forcibly retracting the foreskin).

Further, since the prepuce may be required for repair and, since the concern here is with preserving prepuce, repair of hypospadias, a cosmetic operation, should not be undertaken until the male is of age and able to give his fully informed consent. While urinating from the underside of his penis may be inconvenient, it should be his choice to put up with the inconvenience, rather than having an operation which severs sexually responsive nerves, and leaves him without a fully functioning prepuce during his adult life.

Chordee Without Hypospadias

The penis is bent downwards. This is usually an isolated skin chordee, but may be due to a congenitally short urethra. Circumcision is contraindicated, because the foreskin is needed in the current technique of repair.

Anesthesia

Since all reasonable scientists now recognize that circumcision causes much pain, one would expect the widespread use of anesthesia. This is not happening.

Using anesthesia does not justify performing a circumcision: 1) It usually is not that effective; 2) Harm, and pain, persist long after any anesthesia has worn off.

Complications of Circumcision

One example of a circumcision complication is ulcerative meatitis. Dr. Leonard Marino, in 25 years of practice as a pediatric urologist, stated that 25% of his patients were intact.

None of these ever needed surgery for meatal stenosis, a sequelum of ulcerative meatitis. In contrast, 75 of his circumcised patients required surgery to enlarge the urinary meatus. The accompanying symptoms were dysuria, frequency, hematuria, meatitis, meatal stenosis, urinating more than a single stream. Each patient usually had 4 or more of these symptoms together.[22]

P. Freud writes, "It is astonishing how few articles on this frequent and important disorder have been written and how little the condition is known."[23] It is generally recognized to occur only when the glans is exposed, i.e., in circumcised boys or in intact boys whose prepuce does not completely cover the glans. Ulcers form along the border of the urethral meatus, and the antero-posterior diameter of the meatus is shortened. Urination is very painful and usually requires topical anesthesia to prevent urinary retention. A scar forms after healing. Meatotomy is often required. It is now generally recognized that the narrowing of the meatus is secondary to the thickening of the surface layers of the glans following circumcision.

Psychologic Complications

Settlage has stated, "Concern for the psychologic development and future mental health of the child requires that events in the neonatal as well as any later stage of development be managed in such a way as to keep tension in the child within tolerable limits."[24] During the performance of unanesthetized surgery, these limits may well be exceeded. Preston comments: "One cannot argue that structure and function are intimately related, and at the same time shrug off with equanimity the fretful, circumcised newborn, his glans swollen and cyanotic for three to five days."[25]

The patient has experienced, according to experts, "excruciating pain, the perinatal encoding of his brain with violence, an interruption of maternal-infant bonding, the betrayal of infant trust, and must suffer the risks and effects of permanently altered normal genitalia. In addition, he has lost his basic human right to a sexually intact and functional body."[26]

The Etiology of Circumcision

In case the reader is wondering why all these bizarre excuses have been advanced to permit circumcisions to continue, we offer our best explanation (hypothesis): Circumcision produces circumcisers. The loss of this normal body part is, in some instances, so profound that the person who has lost it is unwilling to admit that anything is wrong. If he becomes a doctor, he may not hesitate to perform circumcisions.

Another hypothesis goes further: Some who have been circumcised cannot stand the idea that someone else might go through life intact. If that person is a doctor, he sees to it. If he is a father, he may insist that his sons be circumcised. A recent analysis stated that the most important factor associated with the decision to circumcise was whether or not the father was circumcised.[27]

We have the greatest admiration for those fathers and those physicians who, while circumcised themselves, say no to having their sons and their patients circumcised.

[1] Wallerstein, E. Circumcision: An American Health Fallacy. New York: Springer Pub Co., 1980

[2] Spock B, Rothenberg MB. Dr Spock's Baby and Child Care 6th Ed New York: Simon & Schuster Inc 1992

[3] Preston EN Circumcision and Genital Hygiene Amer J Dis Child 140: 969, 1986

[4] Jorgensen, ET, Svensson A.The Treatment of Phimosis in Boys, with a potent topical steroid cream. Acta Dermato-Venereologica (Stockholm) 73:55-56, 1993

[5] General Kutuzov quoted in War and Peace by Leo Tolstoy

[6] Cooke JV The etiology and treatment of Ammonia dermatitis of the gluteal region of infants Am J Dis Child 22:481-492,1922

[7] Birley HDL, Walker MM, Luzzi GA, Bell R, Taylor-Robinson D, Byrne M, Renton AM Clinical features and management of recurrent balanitis; association with atopy and genital washing Genitourin Med 69:400-403, 1993

[8] Krueger H, Osborn L Effects of Hygiene Among the Uncircumcised JFam Pract 22:353-355, 1986

[9] Freud P. The Ulcerated Urethral Meatus in Male Children. J Ped. 31:131-141, 1947

[10] Taylor, J. The Prepuce: what exactly is removed by circumcision? Second International Symposium on Circumcision; 1991

[11] Gairdner, D. Fate of the Foreskin Br Med J. 2:1433-1437, 1949

[12] Terris M, Wilson F, Nelson JH. Relation of circumcision to cancer of the cervix. Am J Obstet Gynecol. 117:1056-1066, 1973

[13] Stern E, Neely PM. Cancer of the Cervix in Reference to Circumcision and Marital History. JAMWA 17:739-740, 1962

[14] Wallerstein, E Circumcision: An American Health Fallacy, 1980

[15] Lord, P Personal communication

[16] Escala JM, Rickwood AMK. Balanitis Br J Urol 63:196-197, 1989

[17] Waugh MA Clinical Presentation of Candidal Balanitis—Its Differential Diagnosis and Treatment Chemotherapy 28(Suppl 1):56-60, 1982

[18] Robbins S Pathological Basis of Disease WB Saunders p 1208

[19] Catterall RD, Oates JK. Treatment of Balanitis Xerotica Obliterans with hydrocortisone injections. Brit J Vener. Dis.38:75-77, 1962

[20] Tan HL Foreskin Fallacies and Phimosis Annals Acad Med Singapore 14:626-630, 1985

[21] Rickwood AMK, Hemalatha V, Batcup G, Spitz L. Phimosis in Boys Br J Urol 52:147-150, 1980

[22] Marino LJ An emphatic vote against circumcision Contemp Peds p 14, Nov 1989

[23] Freud P The Ulcerated Urethral Meatus in Male Children J Peds 31:131-141, 1947

[24] Settlage CF. Psychologic Development, in Nelson WE (ed) Textbook of Pediatrics ed 9 WB Saunders p 60, 1969

[25] Preston EN Whither the Foreskin? A Consideration of Routine Neonatal Circumcision JAMA 213:1853-1858, 1970

[26] Milos, MF Macris D. Circumcision A Medical or Human Rights Issue?J Nurse-Midwifery 37:87S-96S, 1992

[27] Brown MS, Brown CA Circumcision decision: prominence of social concerns. Pediatrics 80:215-219, 1987

Notes

1. Lightfoot-Klein, H. *Prisoners of Ritual: An Odyssey into Female Genital Circumcision in Africa*. N.Y.: Haworth Press, 1989.
2. Based on Wallerstein, E. *Circumcision: An American Health Fallacy*. Springer Pub. Co., 1980.
3. *Patient Care Magazine*, March 15, 1978, p 82-85.
4. Gee WF, Ansell JS. *Neonatal Circumcision: A Ten-Year Overview: With Comparison of the Gomco Clamp and the Plastibell Device*. Pediatrics 1976; 58:824-827.
5. Gairdner, D. *The Fate of the Foreskin*. British Medical J. Dec 24, 1949;1433-1437.
6. Based on *Isn't Everybody Circumcised?* and *Intact American Celebrities* by the National Organization of Circumcision Information Resource Centers.
7. Briggs, Ann. *Circumcision: What Every Parent Should Know*. Birth and Parenting Publications, P. O. Box 134, North Garden, VA 22959, $4.95.
8. Based on presentations made at The Second International Symposium on Circumcision by James Bigelow Ph.D.
9. Ibid.
10. Rothenberg, M. *Ending Circumcision in the Jewish Community?* Syllabus of Abstracts, Second International Symposium on Circumcision, April 30, 1991, p. 10.
11. Taken from a report by the National Organization of Circumcision Information Resource Centers.
12. Based on excerpts from *An Appeal to Reason*, National Organization of Circumcision Information Resource Centers.
13. Portions of the remainder of this chapter based on material provided by the National Organization of Circumcision Information Resource Centers.
14. *Redbook*, April 1989, p. 53.
15. *Saturday Evening Post*, July-Aug, 1982, p.6.
16. *San Francisco Examiner*, November 5, 1987, p. E-5.

Selected Medical References

Anand KJS, Hickey PR. Pain and its effects in the human neonate and fetus. *N Engl J Med.* 1987; 317: 1321-1326.
Brigman WE. Circumcision as Child Abuse: The Legal and Constitutional Issues. *J Family Law* 23, no 3, 1984-85.
Cohen HA, Drucker MM, Vainer S, Ashkenasi A, Amir J, Frydman M, Varsano I. Postcircumcision urinary tract infection. Clin Pediatr-Phila 1992 Jun; 31(6):322-4.
Committee on Fetus and Newborn. Report of the Ad Hoc Task Force on Circumcision. Pediatrics 1975; 56:610-611.
Connelly KP, Shropshire LC, Salzberg A. Gastric Rupture Associated with Prolonged Crying in a Newborn Undergoing Circumcision. Clin Pediatr. 1992 Sept; 560-561.
Denniston GC. Circumcision and the Code of Ethics. Humane Health Care International 1996; 12(2):78-80.
Denniston GC. Unnecessary Circumcision. Female Patient 1992; 17:13-14.
Gairdner, D. The Fate of the Foreskin. British Medical J. Dec 24, 1949;1433-1437.
Grimes DA, Routine circumcision of the newborn infant: A reappraisal. Am J Obstet Gynecol 1978; 130:125-129.
Hunter RH. Notes on the development of the prepuce. J. Anat. 1935; 70:68-75.
Kikiros CS, et al. The Response of Phimosis to Local Steroid Application. Ped Surg Intl 1993;8:329-332.
Milos MF, Macris D. Circumcision: A Medical or a Human Rights Issue? J Nurse-Midwifery 1992; 37(2) Suppl: 87S-96S.
Morgan WKC. The rape of the phallus. JAMA 1965; 193:223-4
Preston NE. Whither the Foreskin? A Consideration of Routine Neonatal Circumcision. JAMA 1970; 213:1853-1858.
Prucha ZS. Circumcision? Cutting out the routine cut. Canadian Med Assn J 1980; 122:834.
Rogers MC. Do the Right Thing (Editorial). N Engl J Med 1992; 326:55-56.
Shaw RA, Robertson WO. Routine Circumcision. AM J Dis Child 1963; 106:216-217.
Spock B, Rothenberg MB. Dr Spock's Baby and Child Care. 6th ed. New York: Simon and Schuster, 1992
Svoboda JS, Van Howe RS, Dwyer JG. Informed Consent for Neonatal Circumcision: An Ethical and Legal Conundrum. J. of Contemporary Health Law and Policy 17:61-133
Taddio A, Goldbach M, Ipp M, Stevens B, Koren G. Efect of neonatal circumcision on pain responses during vacc. in boys. Lancet 1995; 345:291-292.
Terris M, Wilson F, Nelson JH. Relation of circumcision to cancer of the cervix. Am J Obstet. Gynecol. 1973; 117:1056-1066.
Wallerstein E. Circumcision: The Uniquely American Medical Enigma. Symposium on Advances in Pediatric Urology, Urologic Clinics of North America 1985; 12:123-132.
Winberg J, Gothefors L, Bollgren I, Herthelius M, Tullus K. The Prepuce: A Mistake of Nature? Lancet 1989; 598-599.

For Information on Circumcision:
In the United States, see page 39-1.
In Australia, NOCIRC P.O. Box 248, Menai, NSW 2234, Australia Fax:+61-2-543-0510
In England, NOCIRC 3 Watlington Rd, Harlow, Essex, CM17 0DX England (0279-419704)

Documenting the Harm:
NOHARMM National Organization to Halt the Abuse and Routine Mutilation of Males, P.O. Box 460795, San Francisco, CA 94146.
Books: *Sex as Nature Intended It,* by Kristen O'Hara with Jeffrey O'Hara. 2001. Turning Point Publications, P.O. Box 486, Hudson, MA 01749. To order, send $19.95 & $3.50 s/h.
You Call This Love? The Real Reason Women Don't Like Sex by Lisa Bisque. 2000. Writers Club Press. Available from iUniverse.com and Amazon.com. $10.95
Questioning Circumcision: A Jewish Perspective and *Circumcision: The Hidden Trauma,* both by Ronald Goldman PhD (888-445-5199).

For those considering restoration:
Read *The Joy of Uncircumcising: Restore your Birthright and Maximize Sexual Pleasure* by Jim Bigelow PhD (see page 20-2).
NORM National Organization of Restoring Men, 3205 Northwood Drive, Suite 209, Concord, CA 94520. Tel 510-827-4077, Fax:510-827-4119

INFANT CIRCUMCISION SURGERY

Note: This surgery is almost always done without anesthesia. The photos presented here were selected from slides of several different actual circumcisions.

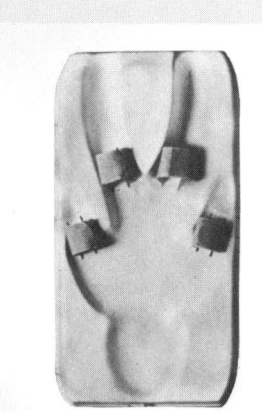

1. Restrain board is used to immobilize newborns during circumcision.

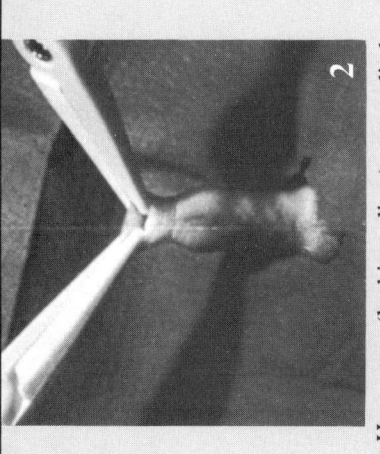

2. Hemostats (locking pliers) are applied to the foreskin (Plastibell technique).

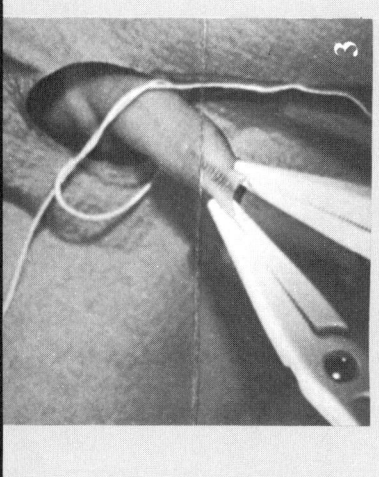

3. Just after the foreskin has been crushed (Plastibell technique).

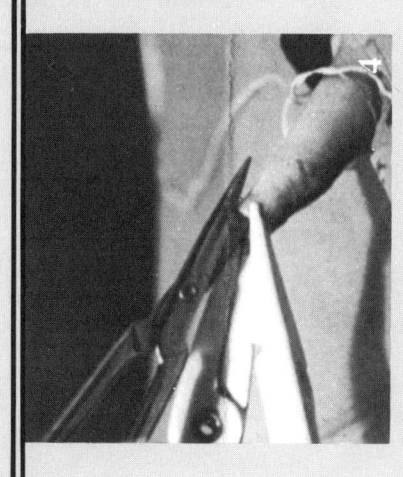

4. Dorsal cut is made in foreskin along the crush line (Plastibell technique).

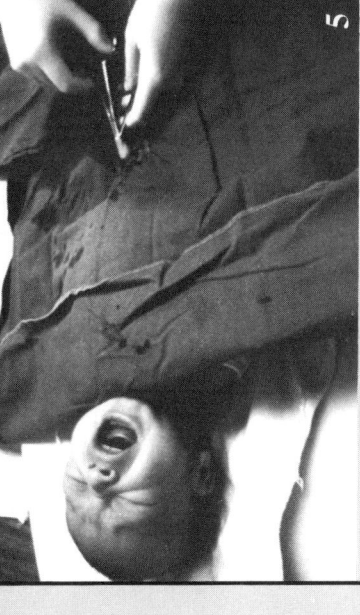

5. Throughout the 5-10 minute surgery, newborns scream, tremble, choke, wail, hold their breath, vomit, agonize...

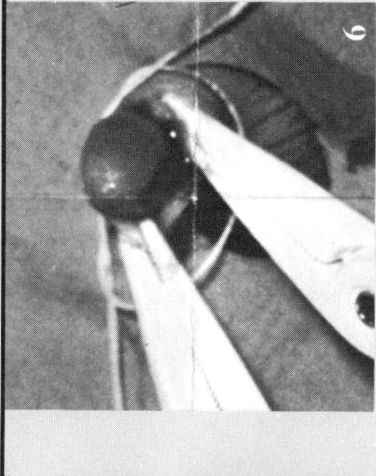

6. Foreskin is peeled back tearing it from the glans (Plastibell technique).

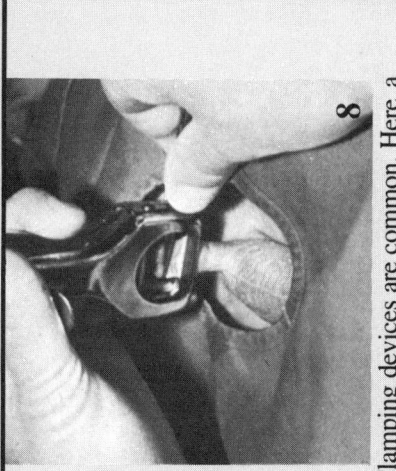

7. Scissors cut off foreskin after bell is inserted and tied (Plastibell technique).

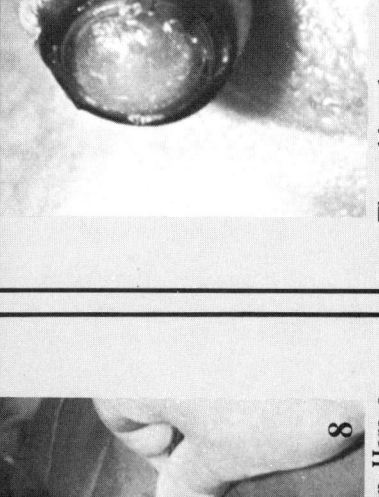

8. Clamping devices are common. Here a Sheldon clamp is used to perform the circumcision.

9. The reddened, exposed, tender, sore glans penis and incision after circumcision.